PASSAGE THROUGH CRISIS

PASSAGE THROUGH CRISIS

Polio Victims and Their Families

Fred Davis

With a New Introduction by the Author

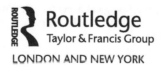

Routledge
Taylor & Francis Group

LONDON AND NEW YORK

Originally Published in 1963 by The Bobbs-Merrill Company, Inc.

Published 1991 by Transaction Publishers

Published 2017 by Routledge
2 Park Square, Milton Park, Abingdon, Oxon OX14 4RN
711 Third Avenue, New York, NY 10017, USA

Routledge is an imprint of the Taylor & Francis Group, an informa business

New material this edition copyright © 1991 by Taylor & Francis.

Library of Congress Catalog Number: 90-31966

Library of Congress Cataloging-in-Publication Data

Davis, Fred, 1925–
    Passage through crisis : polio victims and their families / by
Fred Davis ; with a new introduction by the author.
        p.   cm.
    "Originally published in 1963 by the Bobbs-Merrill Company"—
T.p. verso.
    ISBN 0-88738-853-1
    1. Poliomyelitis—Psychological aspects.   2. Poliomyelitis—
Patients—Family relationships.   I. Title.
RC180.1.D3   1990
362.1'96835—dc20   90-31966
                                                                    CIP

ISBN 13: 978-0-88738-853-8 (pbk)

CONTENTS

INTRODUCTION TO THE TRANSACTION EDITION

In 1957 when I was writing what would appear six years later as *Passage through Crisis,* I found reason at one point to invert a familiar French saying to make it read: *plus c'est la même chose, plus ça change.* This seemed to me at the time, as it still does, an apt characterization of the strong sense of existential continuity that the fourteen families my colleagues and I studied were able to sustain over the many changes, alterations, and dislocations brought about in their lives by their child having contracted paralytic poliomyelitis. Now, thirty and some years later, surveying as best as I can what has happened since in American health care in the way doctors and patients engage each other, I am inclined to revert to the original form of the aphorism: *plus ça change, plus c'est la même chose.*

Let me explain. I do not, of course, mean that everything about American health care practice that ultimately finds its mundane expression in the give-and-take of doctor-patient relations has remained frozen through time. Obviously, a very great deal has changed, so much so as to preclude anything like an adequate review here of the myriad changes, many profound, that have affected one or another aspect of the doctor-patient relationship. These are changes in, to cite the most obvious, medical technology, the administration of physician and hospital practice, health care financing, the general health levels of the population, and the epidemiological patterning of morbidity and mortality including the near disappearance of such "old" diseases as polio itself and the arrival of such dreadful new ones as AIDS and Alzheimer's. In parallel fashion there have been important developments and shifts of emphases in how medical sociologists and other social scientists go about studying health care, in the methodologies they employ, and in the theoretical concepts they bring to bear on their data. I shall want to comment on some of these changes in the course of this introduction. For now, though, let me fix on what seems not to have changed or to have changed very little, namely, the actual encounter of physician and patient and the ensuing exchange between them.

A major finding of *Passage through Crisis* was how very problematic communication was between doctor and patient, although in the particular case of polio the communication was mainly between doctors and the parents of the children who contracted the disease. Contrary to the idealized rational yet humanistic portrait American medicine gave of itself (and in medical sociology where the reigning structural-functionalism of the time was inclined to stand in admiration of that very portrait), my colleagues and I found something quite different. Along with what could be considered a certain amount of frank and straightforward imparting of information to the parents and, clearly, some degree of compassionate concern for them and their stricken children, there was between physician and family also much misunderstanding, manipulation of information, evasiveness, unrealistic expectation, and sheer mistrust. It soon became clear that the physicians (and, in different though complementary ways, nurses and physiotherapists as well) and the families, including the stricken children themselves, held very different "definitions of the situation" with respect to the child's condition and prognosis. These sometimes sharply divergent definitions of medical staff and family persisted well beyond the acute and actively convalescent phases of the disease. The differences were especially apparent in the cases of those families whose children had sustained a more than minimal impairment as a result of the disease. It was as if the then widely presumed guidance-cooperation model of doctor-patient relations (Szasz and Hollander 1956), one in which sensitive and knowledgeable experts are seen to impart accurate information and sound counsel to concerned and trusting clients, had been subverted into what could more nearly be characterized as a manipulation-suspicion model of doctor-patient relations.

Much of *Passage through Crisis* was devoted to analyzing this seemingly anomalous state of affairs. I described there how the divergence in perspectives came about and what consequences this had for the stricken child and for the life of the family. Two facets of this divergence of perspectives were, I felt, particularly salient for understanding the problematic quality of doctor-patient communications. The first, about which I was quite explicit in the book, was that the family's misperceptions and misunderstandings of their child's condition and prospects were in no small part due to the communications of medical treatment personnel themselves: their evasiveness and failure to take sufficient time to explain, and their sometimes defensive, sometimes thoughtless resort to technical language that parents did not understand.

The other aspect of the divergence of perspectives was implicit in much of what I wrote but which I now feel should have been highlighted. It was sociologically incorrect—actually, condescending—to treat the family's divergent perspective as some aberrant, deviant, or culturally benighted version of the "medically authoritative" one, a point of view the reigning medical sociology of the time led one to adopt. Robert Straus (1957) had only recently drawn the telling distinction between sociology *in* medicine and sociology *of* medicine and, immersed as it was in the 1950s' *zeitgeist* of salvation through science, even the sociology *of* medicine, in which I believed my work belonged, tended to reflect viewpoints of a physician-driven sociology *in* medicine. In numerous respects, the family perspective I described represented an authentic embodiment of the natural concerns and conditions of life of the family. As such it qualified for the same sort of existential, if not necessarily medical, legitimation as sociologists were ready to accord the physician perspective with its professionally interested notions of how patients were to think and behave. As Peter Conrad (1984) would observe some twenty years after the publication of *Passage through Crisis*, this was among the very first studies in American medical sociology—and medical sociology as a subdiscipline hardly existed elsewhere in the world then—to take more than incidental account of the patient's perspective and its implications for the illness experiences of people.

A recognition of divergent perspectives and the problems posed thereby for doctor-patient relations, as well as for broad issues of health care generally, was soon to emerge as a focal concern in medical sociology, most notably through the landmark work of Eliot Freidson (1970) in his *Profession of Medicine.* There Freidson examines at length the inherent potential for conflict in the doctor-patient relationship stemming in large part from the very different circumstantial, professional, and life interests each brings to the encounter. The idealized assumption of a true concordance of interest and purpose of doctor and patient can, therefore, be quite mistaken. Rather than potential conflict being dissipated by what many attribute to the patient management skills of the physician (i.e., "bedside manner"), it often festers through the course of treatment. Not infrequently it breaks into the open with heated words and reprimands, though it can also lead, as had been suggested earlier by Balint (1957) and Roth (1963), to a kind of tacit therapeutic negotiation between doctor and patient in which each relinquishes some of what each wants for the sake of holding on to other goals each values.

It is probably fair to characterize this "bringing in of the patient" as constituting a major paradigmatic shift in medical sociology. This was one in which sociologists came to focus less on such physician-framed issues as, for example, patient compliance with regimens, laypersons' medical ignorance, and class variability in health behavior and more on how the lay culture (or, as the phenomenologist phased it, "lebenswelt") of the healthy, sick, and indeterminate intersects with the everyday organized practices of medicine—in sum, the culture of medicine. And because what happens at the intersection came increasingly to be seen in terms of a divergence or conflict or, at very least, a melding of perspectives, the medical sociologist could begin to fashion analytic schemes and accounts less dependent for their interpretative validity, their explanatory sense of rightness, on the professional interests and ideologies of organized medicine. The easy, comforting assumption of this era of scientific medicine that "doctor knew best" about *all* things bearing on health and illness had ended in medical sociology as it was soon to end in health affairs generally.

Since the 1970s this paradigmatic shift in medical sociology, of which *Passage through Crisis* was, perhaps, something of a harbinger, has been greatly strengthened by a number of converging sociolinguistic, semiotic, structuralist, and poststructuralist approaches. (See, for example, Anspach 1988, Fisher and Todd 1983, Mishler 1984, Strong 1979, Turner 1987, and Waitzkin 1989.) All of these underscore in one fashion or another the profound degree to which the "discourse" of medicine, either as articulated or, more salient yet, as enacted in the everyday encounters of physicians and patients, structures the orienting and operative realities of the parties to the transaction. Simultaneously, it both sustains and reproduces the power relations and social control practices obtaining between them. Thus, it is more than attitude, information, knowledge, and good or ill will which account for the many misadventures and, contrariwise, successes of physician-patient encounters. Before all else it resides in the underlying terms of the relationship or, if you will, in the deep taken-for-granted experiential constitution by which each knows, sees, and talks to the other: you *doctor,* I *patient.*

That something so fundamental, so encapsulating as not to be seen, could account for the many difficulties of communication and comprehension experienced by the families we studied is an insight that all but eluded me in *Passage through Crisis.* The book does speak of the great power discrepancy of physician and patient and of its significance for what parents came to believe (and misbelieve) concerning the child's condition. But the myriad, interwoven ways—in talk, inflection, gesture, demeanor, clothing, time management, spatial placement, etc.—by which this power realizes itself, as it simultaneously sustains a discourse of physician dominance (see Foucault 1980), was only glancingly apprehended by me. It has, to its credit, been left to a succeeding generation of students to capture and formulate.

It has, though, been a good deal more than theoretical developments in medical sociology that has served to uncover the socially *constructed* character of the physician-client exchange and of the discourse that cloaks it in a taken-for-granted, at times seemingly preordained, naturalness. Beginning in the mid to late 1960s there began to emerge on the American scene, no doubt influenced in some part by the civil rights and minority-group struggles of that decade, a profusion of health-related self-help groups. Mushrooming in the manner of some vast social movement, these came in time to cover the gamut of human disabilities and misfortunes including the addictions; biologically damaging genetic anomalies; disabling diseases such as multiple sclerosis, stroke, and Parkinson's; postoperative disfigurements associated, for example, with mastectomies, ileostomies, and colostomies; the terminal phases of such conditions as cancer and kidney disease; and the distress of family members whose kin suffered from one or another of the above or possibly some other condition overlooked in this far-from-exhaustive listing. What is significant about such self-help groups, quite apart from the help and support their members give each other, is that their very coming into being highlights the vast terrain of human worry, emotion, practical concern, and interpersonal disturbance left unattended and unalleviated by the institutions of medicine *per se*. Not that these would prove altogether tractable for medicine or, for that matter, any organized professional practice. But inasmuch as they do fall into that broad domain of health and illness that medicine claims exclusively for itself, the concerns and preoccupations dealt with in such groups bring into question many of the terms and tendencies of the physician-client and hospital-patient relationships—as has the emergence of a more active health consumerism (Reeder 1972). Developments of this sort usher into awareness the socially constructed particularities of these relationships. In so doing they suggest possibilities for revision and reconstruction.

Such has been evidenced in perhaps the most profound manner imaginable in the instance of the disease AIDS since its appearance in the 1980s. Due in no small part to the organization and political militancy of Gay community groups and associations such as Act-Up (Aids Coalition to Unleash Power), some very important changes are being effected in doctor-patient relations and in numerous hitherto established, hardly ever questioned, much less challenged, health policies and practices in America.

To make it possible for persons who have contracted the AIDS virus to secure potentially beneficial drug therapies more easily, federal policies regulating the testing, approval, and licensing of new drugs have been significantly modified. Similarly, to insure that the privacy, civil rights, and employment of those infected by the AIDS virus (as well as that of their sexual partners and associates) are not violated or unduly compromised, in cities with large Gay and intravenous drug-using populations strong safeguards have been instituted against the release of information by doctors and public health authorities that would identify HIV carriers and those already ill from the disease. Notwithstanding the widespread stigmatization still directed at homosexuals and drug users in American society, these safeguards, ironically, have in the main proven more stringent than those imposed in the past for such communicable and/or sexually transmitted diseases as tuberculosis, hepatitis B, syphilis, and gonorrhea. In its concern for minimizing the discrimination, ostracism, and outright abuse its members might encounter as a result of the AIDS epidemic, the Gay community has been able, often with the vocal support of AIDS researchers and leading medical figures, to modify in important respects what formerly was viewed as a taken-for-granted public health right—indeed, at times a positive obligation—namely, to advise and notify persons at risk due to having been in intimate contact with a known carrier of a serious communicable disease (Mueller 1989).

More important than these statutory and policy changes are the alterations the disease is bringing about, in part due perhaps to the drama attached to its intractability, in the interaction of doctors and AIDS patients and, accordingly, in the very nature of their relationship. Unwilling to rely in some passive and acquiescent manner on the putative expertise of the physician, AIDS patients, their friends, and families have become extremely active in their own treatment and critical of that dispensed them by medical authorities. Newspaper reports in late 1988 tell of AIDS patients and their friends accessing via their computers medical data bases for the latest research reports on experimental drugs being developed for the treatment of AIDS. The findings from such reports would often be used to challenge the pronouncements and prescriptions of their physicians. Physicians were reported as stating that the experience of dealing with patients more knowledgeable than themselves about some critical aspect of their treatment was altogether novel. This could not but help cast the doctor-patient relationship on a plane very different from that to which they were accustomed.

In their classic 1956 paper on different styles of doctor-patient interaction, Szasz and Hollander delineated what they term a mutually participative model. They went on to note, however, that despite its many therapeutic virtues (the humanizing effect of reducing social distance between doctor and patient being a principal one) the mutually participative mode was far from the most prevalent form of doctor-patient interaction. When found at all in medical practice, it tended to occur, though rarely at that, in such relatively peripheral and problematic areas of medicine as psychiatry and rehabilitative medicine. Clearly, though, some such model is now being realized in important measure in the medical treatment of AIDS. Of course, it cannot be presumed that similar shifts are occurring to nearly the same extent in other quarters of medical practice. Still, the greater sophistication, health awareness, and educational attainment of major segments of the American population since the Szasz and Hollander article and the writing of *Passage through Crisis* give reason to hope that the new model of doctor-patient relations arising from the tragic ground of AIDS may in the period ahead evolve in other areas of medical practice and health care as well. This is in small part already happening with the growth since the later 1960s of a consumerist ideology in the field of health affairs (Reeder 1972). In general, the increased activism of patients, their demands to be kept better informed, and their reluctance to remain dumbly acquiescent in the face of "expert" pronouncements are part and parcel of the broader, albeit uneven, movements of democratization and deprofessionalization occurring in health care fields over the past two decades.

The impact of AIDS on medical practice and health care touches on yet another interesting turn in medical sociological studies, as well as other social science and humanistic writing on health and disease, since *Passage through Crisis* first appeared. I refer to a subtler appreciation by scholars of the deep metaphoric significance certain diseases hold for the *zeitgeist* of an era and for the cultural milieu animating it. Again, in *Passage through Crisis* this was a connection more felt than amplified. In the book I point, for example, to how very much the gradient structuring of the physiotherapeutic regime prescribed for the convalescing children drew on a Protestant-inspired moral calculus of stepwise, dedicated effort in pursuit of worthy distant goals. Earlier, in the chapter on "The Crisis Experience," I relate how the the child's having been stricken with polio was experienced by many of the parents as a kind of "betrayal of the American dream." For the most part, however, the range and richness of the cultural reverberations, echoes, and retorts emanating from the intersection of disease and historical consciousness was to be left for others to plumb, albeit from quite different perspectives. Most notable in this connection are the works of Dubos (1959), Sontag (1978, 1988), and, more closely tied to medical sociology *per se* than either, Herzlich and Pierret (1987). With much sensitivity these writers explore the ways a disease, its symptomatic profile, the anxieties it generates, the populations it strikes, and the dramaturgy of public efforts to combat it resonate with the deepest chords of a culture and the historical epoch.

Thanks to their work I see more clearly now how deeply embedded the social phenomenology of paralytic poliomyelitis was in the American mood of hope, in the scientific innocence and unquestioning faith in the future that prevailed during the fifteen to twenty year period following the Second World War. The symbolic configuration of polio in the public's imagination reflected this in numerous ways. It was primarily a disease of children, persons least meriting ill fortune and upon whom altruism could be showered unstintingly. Moreover, by mid-century polio had come to strike disproportionately large numbers of children from middle class families, that is, families whose life-style most vividly displayed core American values. Drawing on a faith in science's ability to overcome, within a foreseeable future if not immediately, nearly all misfortune and adversity, concern over the disease had given birth to a massive voluntary public effort, the Mother's March of Dimes. Religious zeal coupled to the most advanced devices of modern fund-raising raised massive amounts of money to underwrite the research that would vanquish the disease, as indeed largely came to pass by the mid 1950s with the advent of the Salk and Sabin vaccines. The disease had found its icon in the immensely popular and revered figure of the late president, Franklin D. Roosevelt. Himself a victim of polio, he had successfully led the country through a great depression and global war from which America emerged as the world's preeminent power. And, just as science, in the form of the atom bomb, had finally subdued America's World War II enemies, so would it, one knew instinctively, vanquish the dreaded enemy poliomyelitis. Despite the human costs in crippling and death polio had already exacted and would continue to exact, the metaphor of a just war from which America would emerge triumphant suffused nearly every facet of the public's consciousness of poliomyelities.

Today AIDS stands in vivid contrast to this imagery and signals how far America has moved from the postwar era of earnest hope in and naive celebration of the fruits of scientific discovery. Whereas a spirit of community voluntarism marked the struggle against polio (Sills 1957), something more akin to political activism is at the forefront of organized efforts to treat and find a cure for AIDS (Shilts 1988). As for root metaphors one need not, perhaps, go as far as Susan Sontag (1988), who sees in AIDS an evocation of that diffuse foreboding of global annihilation (be it nuclear, ecological, or demographic) that has come to hover over humankind since the fading of the early postwar "better things for better living through chemistry" euphoria. (More often now chemistry *is* the culprit!) Well short of so cataclysmic a vision it is at once evident that the dramaturgy of AIDS plays to a very different consciousness and societal configuration. As Sontag herself in a less apocalyptic vein notes, it speaks to limits, to constraints, the bridling of impulse, the curbing of freedoms, and the abjuring of permissiveness—all of this clothed in an easily summonable morality play of Jehovistic retribution visited on a modern analogue of Sodom and Gomorrah. Scientific rescue seems less certain, too. Notwithstanding some four decades of major advances in medical knowledge and technology, the hope of finding a cure for AIDS or some sure means for preventing its spread is met with a good deal of pessimism. This, too, stands in sharp relief to the optimism following World War II regarding the possible discovery of an antidote for the then equally baffling polio virus. Like the bewildering, seemingly contradictory environmental threats to earth's atmosphere (holes in the ozone layer alongside dangerous levels of ozone due to the greenhouse effect), every new finding concerning AIDS and its transmission seems soon confounded by exceptions, complications, and alternate strains of the HIV that behave differently.

When a work such as this is republished some twenty-seven years after its initial appearance, it seems only natural to want to look back on how it was received at the time. Had reviewers grasped its main points? Were they fair in their appraisal of the book's significance?

Authors given this rare opportunity, as I am here, are notorious for bemoaning the "misunderstandings" and "distortions" book reviewers are alleged to have inflicted on their work. Drawing on hindsight's wisdom they justify and "make clear" what they themselves probably failed to make clear in the first place.

No such stratagems, I am pleased to say, are required in the case of *Passage through Crisis,* although the reviews themselves are not without a certain historic interest in light of what has happened in sociology over the past quarter century. Actually, the book was, with one partial exception, quite favorably reviewed in the professional journals and, as these things go, enjoyed fairly brisk sales over the fourteen or so years it was kept in print. Reviewers spoke favorably of the work's clear and naturalistic style, its insights, and its conceptual clarity. Two of them grasped at once what subsequently, as the book entered the working literature of medical sociology, came to be viewed as its most telling contribution, that is, the delineation of the disjunction of physician and family perspectives and medicine's failure to compensate for this in any therapeutically beneficent way. No reviewer was troubled by the fact the book dealt with paralytic poliomyelitis, a disease that by the time of the book's appearance had been all but eradicated in North America and the rest of the developed world. The implications of the study were understood correctly to lie well beyond any specific disease *per se.* The social psychology of illness experiences and the impact of illness on family organization and functioning were duly noted by reviewers as the book's essential topics.

Considering the quantitative empiricism that dominated the

sociology of the time—sample surveys were the ruling methodology and large samples of meticulous representativeness were thought the royal road to scientific truth—reviewers were remarkably forgiving of what one of them warned readers was a mere "N of 14." Even this reviewer, however, held that the book's sociologically sophisticated treatment of an important problem justified setting aside usual statistical criteria. I was especially pleased with the review because, as is not altogether untrue today, nearly any qualitative microsociological work was likely to be summarily dismissed for the "unrepresentativeness of its findings." Qualitative, ethnographically oriented researchers such as myself lacked even a language with which to challenge the positivist criticism that was virtually certain to be directed at works like *Passage through Crisis*. Such present-day epistemologies as deconstructionism and discourse analysis for rebutting empiricist strictures (see Gusfield 1981, Marcus and Fisher 1986) were hardly available at the time. The best one could do was to make apologetic noises about how "small sample, in-depth studies" might generate the hypotheses for the more definitive, large scale, quantitative studies one hoped would follow. (The very terms of defense were clothed in the reigning language of positivist epistemology!) The careful reader will note that *Passage through Crisis* itself is not altogether free of such defensiveness. Still, much as I encountered this sort of criticism from some of those who were to become familiar with the work, it was reassuring not to have to confront it in journal reviews. In any event, I would hope that the favorable reception accorded *Passage through Crisis* might have encouraged other students to feel somewhat less apprehensive about their "small N's" and more sanguine of the conceptual possibilities accruing to small scale, in-depth qualitative studies.

This reprinting of *Passage through Crisis* would not have come to pass were it not for a chance meeting with David Mechanic and several of his medical sociology graduate students at the August 1988 Atlanta meetings of the American Sociological Association. The students spoke to me of their admiration of the work and of the difficulty they had in obtaining even library copies of the book. They asked whether I had given any thought to having it republished. In truth, I had not, or at least not until that moment. Soon thereafter Mechanic brought the matter to the attention of Irving Louis Horowitz, publisher of Transaction at Rutgers University, who forthwith wrote me a warm letter of interest and encouragement in having the book republished. It is, then, with a deep sense of gratitude I wish to thank David Mechanic, his students, and Irving Louis Horowitz for having so palpably revived the life of *Passage through Crisis.*

REFERENCES

Anspach, Renee R. 1988. "Notes on the Sociology of Medical Discourse: The Language of Case Presentation." *Journal of Health and Social Behavior* 29, No. 4:357–375.

Balint, Michael. 1957. *The Doctor, His Patient and the Illness.* New York: International Universities Press.

Conrad, Peter. 1984. "Classics Revisited." *Disability and Chronic Disease Quarterly* 4, No. 3 (July):20–21.

Dubos, Rene. 1959. *Mirage of Health.* Garden City, N. Y.: Doubleday.

Fisher, Sue, and Alexandra D. Todd, eds. 1983. *The Social Organization of Doctor-Patient Communication.* Washington, D.C.: Center for Applied Linguistics.

Foucault, Michel. 1980. *Power/Knowledge: Selected Interviews and Other Writings.* New York: Pantheon.

Freidson, Eliot. 1970. *Profession of Medicine.* New York: Dodd, Mead.

Gusfield, Joseph R. 1981. *The Culture of Public Problems.* Chicago: University of Chicago Press.

Herzlich, Claudine, and Janine Pierret. 1987. *Illness and Self in Society.* Baltimore: The Johns Hopkins University Press.

Marcus, George E., and Michael M. J. Fisher. 1986. *Anthropology As Cultural Critique.* Chicago: University of Chicago Press.

Mishler, Elliot G. 1984. *The Discourse of Medicine.* Norwood, N.J.: Ablex.

Mueller, Mary Rose. 1989. "California's Proposition 64: A Sociological Study of its Controversies and Ironies." Unpublished paper.

Reeder, Leo G. 1972. "The Patient-Client as a Consumer." *Journal of Health and Social Behavior* 13, No. 4:406–412.

Roth, Julius. 1963. *Timetables*. Indianapolis: Bobbs-Merrill.

Shilts, Randy. 1988. *And the Band Played On: Politics, People and the Aids Epidemic*. New York: St. Martin's.

Sills, David L. 1957. *The Volunteers, Means and Ends in a National Organization*. Glencoe, I.L.: Free Press.

Sontag, Susan. 1978. *Illness As Metaphor*. New York: Farrar, Straus and Giroux.

Sontag, Susan. 1988. *AIDS and Its Metaphors*. New York: Farrar, Straus and Giroux.

Straus, Robert. 1957. "The Nature and Status of Medical Sociology." *American Sociological Review* 22:200–204.

Strong, P. M. 1979. *The Ceremonial Order of the Clinic*. London: Routledge & Kegan Paul.

Szasz, Thomas S., and Mark H. Hollander. 1956. "A Contribution to the Philosophy of Medicine." *A. M. A. Archives of Internal Medicine* 97: 585–592.

Turner, Bryan S. 1987. *Medical Power and Social Knowledge*. London: Sage.

Waitzkin, Howard. 1989. "A Critical Theory of Medical Discourse." *Journal of Health and Social Behavior* 30, No. 2:220–239.

ACKNOWLEDGMENTS

This study derives from an interdisciplinary research carried out during the years 1953-57 at the Psychiatric Institute of the University of Maryland, in Baltimore. That undertaking, known as the Polio Project, was supported largely by a grant from the National Foundation (then the National Foundation for Infantile Paralysis). The preparation of an earlier and more extended version of the present volume (*Polio in the Family, A Study of Crisis and Family Process,* Unpublished Doctoral Dissertation, Department of Sociology, University of Chicago, 1958) was made possible by a training grant from the National Institutes of Health, United States Public Health Service.

I am, of course, greatly indebted to these organizations, but even more so to my former colleagues in the Polio Project, without whose collaboration in the collection of data the present book could never have materialized. They are Joseph S. Bierman, the late Jacob E. Finesinger, Martin Gorten, Joseph Greenblum, Harvey A. Robinson, Arthur Silverstein, and Toba Tahl. Although their work and thought are reflected on every page of this book, they cannot be held responsible for whatever errors of interpretation or construction may have found their way into it. I hope that they will be tolerant of my failure to credit them individually for the many, now hopelessly intermingled ideas, insights, and findings that originated with one or another of them.

At various times since the work's inception, friends and colleagues have offered valuable suggestions, criticisms, and, most important, fresh interpretative approaches to the data. In particular, I wish to thank Renée Fox, Erving Goffman, Sheldon Messinger, Stephen Richardson, Julius Roth, and Anselm Strauss. The final product would have been a much poorer thing without their excellent counsel. No formal acknowledgment can adequately express my gratitude to my wife, Marcella, for her patience, sympathetic criticism, and encouragement.

Finally, I welcome this opportunity to express publicly my appreciation to the fourteen families who are the subjects of this study. The kindness and good humor with which they consistently received my colleagues and me, despite the strains of this major ordeal in their lives, were generous in the extreme.

FRED DAVIS

San Francisco, California
January 1962

PASSAGE THROUGH CRISIS

Polio Victims and Their Families

THIS

Chapter 1. Introduction

book is an account of the social-psychological impact of a serious illness on fourteen children and their families. The illness is spinal paralytic poliomyelitis; the subjects are the members of fourteen urban families in which a child contracted the disease, was hospitalized for an extended period, and returned home—nearly always—with a physical handicap. The families were first seen during 1954-55, immediately prior to the full-scale introduction of the Salk anti-polio vaccine, when many facts and rumors were being circulated about the vaccine but when parents could not as yet procure it for their children.

At time of onset of the disease, the eight boys and six girls ranged in age from four to twelve. The primary site of paralytic involvement for all was the lower extremities, although with some, other portions of the body (e.g., abdomen, forearm, fingers) were also affected. Upon admission to the hospital, all the children but one had been diagnosed as either moderately or severely paralyzed. The children came from predominantly working class families, there being only four in which the parents could be classified as either lower-middle or middle class. All the families were white and native-born; the ethnic backgrounds of a majority of them were what is loosely termed

Protestant Anglo-Saxon. Of the remaining families, two were Jewish, two Catholic, and two of mixed Protestant-Catholic affiliation.[1]

The research design of the study was longitudinal; that is, the same families were seen at regular intervals, beginning within a week of the child's admission to a general hospital and terminating some fifteen months after his discharge from a convalescent hospital. In general, this encompassed an 18- to 24-month span in which the research team maintained repeated contact with the child, his parents, and the hospital personnel charged with his treatment and care.

A variety of medical, psychological, and sociological methods and techniques was utilized in studying the families.[2] From the data gathered it was possible to chart and compare reactions, to note changes over periods of time, and, in general, to trace in developmental terms the adjustments of the families to the altered life circumstances occasioned by the child's illness and its aftermath.

POLIO: DISEASE AND POPULAR SYMBOL

Until the first successful mass administration of the Salk anti-polio vaccine, in 1955, poliomyelitis enjoyed the infamous distinction of being the only remaining serious epidemic disease in the Western world. Its over-all incidence had never been especially high compared, for example, to that of such nonepidemic diseases as tuberculosis, heart disease, and cancer, but, as an epidemic disease, it tended to strike a whole community suddenly and unpredictably, leaving in its wake much malaise, crippling, and death, particularly among children and youth.[3] Thus, whereas the mean annual incidence of the disease for the whole of the United States in 1940-47 was but 10 per 100,000 population, in Minnesota during this same period it was 22. In such notorious epidemics as those in New York in 1931 and Berlin in 1947 the rates were 59 and 76, respectively. But even these figures fail to convey the peculiar notoriety that the disease had acquired prior to

[1] For a listing of the families, their composition, and their major social characteristics, see Appendix B, pp. 188-90.

[2] For a detailed account of the design and methods of the research, see Appendix A, pp. 181-86.

[3] The pathology and sequelae of paralytic poliomyelitis are described on pp. 48-80.

the recent discovery of effective preventive measures. For, since polio is a disease affecting children primarily, the age-specific incidence rates always ran markedly higher in the younger age groups than in the population at large. Thus, in the New York and Berlin epidemics, the specific rates for the highly susceptible five-to-nine-year-old group were 226 and 360, respectively.[4] Even in an "average" pre-1955 year, the incidence rate among children in this age group living in metropolitan areas of the United States was approximately 50.

Epidemiological statistics alone, however, cannot account for the awe and dread with which polio had come to be regarded or for the very special consideration and mass sympathy extended to its victims.[5] Certainly, in a child-centered culture such as ours, some of this feeling can be attributed to the fact that polio is so predominantly a disease of childhood and early adolescence. The crippling it often caused would also seem to be an important factor, although it should be noted that, even in fairly serious polio epidemics, nonparalytic cases generally outnumbered paralytic cases ten to twenty-five times.[6] In ways difficult to ascertain, the apparent (by no means well-documented) tendency of the disease prior to 1955 to exact a disproportionately great toll among children in the middle and upper socioeconomic classes may also have influenced public apprehension.[7]

[4] T. Sabin, "Epidemiologic Patterns of Poliomyelitis in Different Parts of the World," in *Poliomyelitis: Papers and Discussions Presented at the First International Poliomyelitis Conference,* Philadelphia: Lippincott, 1949, pp. 3-33.

[5] On the extent of such public concern see J. Clausen, M. Seidenfeld, and L. Deasy, "Parent Attitudes Toward Participation in Polio Vaccine Trials," in E. Gartley Jaco, ed., *Patients, Physicians and Illness,* Glencoe, Ill.: Free Press, 1958, pp. 124-25.

[6] P. M. Stimson, "Poliomyelitis Aphorisms," *Journal of Pediatrics,* XLIV (June, 1954), 608.

[7] Virologists account for the differential social class incidence of the disease prior to 1955 by pointing out that, because of the comparatively unhygienic surroundings and practices of poorer families, children from this stratum were more likely to have been exposed early in life to mild strains of the disease virus than were middle or upper class children. As a result they developed resistant antibodies that stood them in good stead when they were later exposed to the virulent strains of polio virus that would accompany epidemics. Since 1955, however, the pattern of social class incidence of the disease has, if anything, been reversed. Middle and upper class families have availed themselves of the Salk and Sabin vaccines in proportionately greater numbers than have working class families; the small remaining incidence of the disease, therefore, tends to be concentrated in the working classes.

What most distinguished poliomyelitis from other equally severe and prevalent diseases, however, is that it had been made the object of one of the largest and most highly organized voluntary movements in American history. Since the early thirties, the National Foundation for Infantile Paralysis, with its many fund-raising, educational, welfare, research, and promotional activities, had touched and penetrated in one fashion or another almost every community and social grouping in the nation.[8] It served as the model for a host of other national voluntary associations dedicated to the prevention, treatment, and cure of such diseases as mental illness, cancer, epilepsy, heart disease, and muscular dystrophy. A major factor in the growth and accomplishments of the National Foundation—culminating in Enders' laboratory isolation of the polio virus and Salk's development of the anti-polio vaccine—was the figure of Franklin D. Roosevelt, whose service to his country despite his long and arduous experience with paralytic polio not only inspired his fellow sufferers but also publicized the work and aims of the foundation to the nation.

It is not surprising, therefore, that of the many critical diseases which afflict man, polio had come to occupy a pre-eminent—and, according to some, an exaggerated—place in the awareness, sympathy, and philanthropy of the American people.[9] By the time of the development of the Salk vaccine it had emerged in popular thought as more than a sometimes crippling disease of children; it was regarded as a powerful symbol of blind, devastating, and uncontrollable misfortune whose victims were specially entitled to the support and good will of the community.

POLIO AS AN OBJECT OF SOCIOLOGICAL STUDY

I cite this background for two reasons: first, for what it may convey to the reader of the "polio *zeitgeist*" surrounding the crisis reaction of the 14 families to be described here; and second, as a means of intro-

[8] For an excellent analysis of the history, organization, and program of the foundation and the movement it fathered, see David L. Sills, *The Volunteers: Means and Ends in a National Organization*, Glencoe, Ill.: Free Press, 1957.

[9] For a possible explanation of the "epidemiologically biased" public concern with polio, see O. Simmons, "Implications of Social Class for Public Health," in Jaco, ed., *op. cit.*, p. 108.

ducing, and attempting to answer, certain basic questions regarding the study that the reader may, quite properly, feel impelled to raise. Of what value is it, one might ask, to report on the experiences of families with a disease that appears to be well on its way toward becoming extinct? Moreover, is not the train of medical and social events set in motion by this disease so unique as to offer no basis for increasing our understanding of what happens in families stricken by other serious illnesses, much less by nonmedical crises of an equally disruptive kind? Finally, even assuming that certain meaningful parallels can be adduced in these connections, what broader theoretical purposes, if any, does such a study serve? I shall briefly consider each of these questions.

As regards the first question, it should be noted that although polio may well be "on its way" toward becoming an extinct disease, at least in the medically advanced parts of the world, this millenium has not yet arrived. Despite a markedly reduced incidence since 1955,[10] a sizable number of persons, mostly children, still contracts the paralytic variety of the disease. Much of the remaining incidence can no doubt be explained by the failure of these persons to avail themselves of the number of Salk-vaccine inoculations necessary to ensure a high degree of protection, but a significant residual proportion of it—recently estimated at 29 percent—can be attributed to the less than total effectiveness of the vaccine itself.[11] (Whether other newly developed preventive measures, such as the Sabin oral vaccine, will prove more effective has yet to be definitely demonstrated.) In any event, it is probable that for some years to come a considerable number of children will continue to contract the disease and be handicapped as a result. From a practical standpoint, therefore, a systematic account of some of the numerous problems experienced by families in which this happens would seem to be of value.

[10] Compared to an average annual incidence of 10 per 100,000 population prior to 1955, the rates for the United States as a whole in 1957, 1958, and 1959 were 3.2, 3.3, and 4.8 respectively. *Metropolitan Life Statistical Bulletin,* XLI, 9 (September, 1960), 6-8.

[11] Of all paralytic cases reported for the United States during 1959, 29 percent had received three or more properly spaced doses of Salk vaccine. Of these inoculated victims, approximately 65 percent were aged 5 to 19 years (U.S. Department of Health, Education and Welfare, *Poliomyelitis Surveillance Report: 1960,* Communicable Disease Center, Atlanta, Ga., 1960).

Does the study have relevance beyond the specific patterning of events comprising paralytic polio as such? I believe that it does. In analyzing the relatively long-term involvement of 14 families in the social vicissitudes caused by this particular disruptive experience, we are perforce inquiring into such generalized matters as the perception of sudden crises by families, the effects on the family unit of prolonged hospitalization (or other separation from the home) of family members, problems in doctor-patient communication, and the identity stresses arising from alterations in the bodily self. Although it is true that the precise manifestations of these events and problems will vary with the nature of the crisis or family situation, there are enough structural and processual similarities to contribute to our knowledge of general conditions, provided that the generic properties of these various crises are so delineated as to make comparisons possible.

Finally, as regards the theoretical relevance of the study, we might mention the continuing need in sociology for concrete empirical analyses of what Talcott Parsons has termed the exchanges between major social subsystems in our society. Among these subsystems would certainly be numbered the family and the hospital. Not only are these engaged in frequent and highly salient exchanges, but each, as we shall see, is also greatly implicated in the stability, the decision-making, and the problem-solving of the other.[12] Regardless, then, of the nature of the illness or which family member is afflicted, a study of the complex social relations brought into being by hospitalization can shed light on such theoretically relevant issues as the boundary-defining and maintaining properties of the two subsystems; the points at which their respective needs, normative orientations, and values support and conflict with each other; and the accommodations that each, following its own distinctive organizational bent, can and cannot make to the other. No single study so limited in scope as this one can presume to provide exhaustive answers to such questions; but it can call attention to a range of considerations that need to be taken into account if fruitful theory is to develop in this area.

[12] A leading theoretical statement on the social dimensions of the family-hospital relationship, certain portions of which are disputed in later chapters of this book, is T. Parsons and R. Fox, "Illness, Therapy, and the Modern Urban American Family," in E. Gartley Jaco, ed., *op. cit.*, pp. 234-45.

SCOPE AND EMPHASES OF THE STUDY

I regard this as a naturalistic study. It neither focuses on a single aspect of the family's experience with the child's illness and its aftermath nor does it try, as does much present-day sociological research, to test a series of preformulated hypotheses on highly delimited and analytically refined facets of the experience. Finally, because of the small number of subjects involved, this study cannot be viewed as a sample survey of the ways in which families in general react when one of their children is struck by polio.

A much more descriptive and inductive tendency characterizes this work. I have attempted to describe and analyze certain experiences common to the families studied as they moved from one set of conditions to the next—the onset of the child's illness, its diagnosis as polio, the child's hospitalization, the course of his treatment, his discharge from the hospital, and his reincorporation into the family setting. Both in time and in depth, this sequence encompassed a very broad and varied range of life experience for the families that could not possibly be fully described in so small a volume as this. In the six chapters that follow, therefore, I shall deal mainly with the natural history of the unfolding of the polio crisis experience in the family (Chapter 2); the families' conceptions of the disease and the recovery process; alterations in these conceptions as a result of the hospital experience and interaction with treatment personnel; and the strains, communication problems, and clashes of perspectives to which this experience and interaction gave rise (Chapter 3); the perspectives on recovery developed by different families following the child's return home and the relationship of these to the severity of the child's residual handicap (Chapter 4); the effects of the child's illness and hospitalization on family functioning, both during the period of his separation from the family setting and during his subsequent reincorporation into it (Chapter 5); the problems in identity posed for child and family by his newly acquired status as a handicapped person and the major adjustive stratagems they employed (Chapter 6); and a summary discussion of certain of the broader implications of the study for continuing and emerging issues in sociology (Chapter 7).

Throughout the book, three major themes recur. For the moment these may be designated as emergence, continuity of identity, and clash of interests between hospital and home.

Emergence

Emergence has to do mainly with the pacing, quality, and development of the families' reactions over a period of time to the many novel conditions and events occasioned by the child's illness. The summary concept of emergence is used here in opposition to the more familiar sociological notion of inherence. That is to say, the reactions displayed by the families were not in any strict sense "determined" by the objective events themselves; nor, on the other hand, can it be said that they issued mainly from any personality characteristics, attitudes, or interpersonal configurations pre-existent and latent in the makeup of each family. Instead, the reactions of the families can best be described in terms of an ongoing developmental process—an improvisatory "building up," as it were, in which each new event posed new problems that in turn generated a trial-and-error search for new interpretations and definitions of the situation. This search resulted not only in perceptual modifications of the existent situation, but in unwitting re-evaluations of relevant past and impending situations as well.[13] Thus, the actual undergoing of the process set its own conditions for further action, the conditions themselves being an existential amalgam of previously emergent responses and events. This process, we would hold, defies simple causal reduction to some original state of immanence or fixed set of determining events. Although it is possible to detect, *post hoc,* certain regularities in the process, this is not to say that its end-states are wholly contained in its beginnings.

Continuity of Identity

The foregoing remarks raise the question how, in view of such flux and indeterminancy, the families were able—as, we shall show, they were—to maintain some sense of stability and sameness in their lives.

[13] A seminal presentation of this approach to the analysis of experience is that of George H. Mead, *The Philosophy of the Present,* Chicago: Open Court, 1932.

Why did they not become alienated, disorganized, or otherwise detached from their historic sense of who and what they were? We hold, paradoxically, that continuity of identity was preserved mainly as a result of the emergent character of the ongoing adjustment process—with its redefinitions, re-evaluations, and retrospective reconstructions. Through this process the past was made to fit the present, so to speak. This realignment then set the stage for a subjectively more congruent response to what in the actual past had been, but no longer was, a wholly unanticipated future.

Consider, for example, but a few of the many altered situations that most of the families came to confront in time: a changed balance of rewards and punishments in the disciplining of children in the family, both during and after the sick child's hospitalization; hospital-induced changes in the sick child's interaction with his siblings; the negative social meanings attached to his handicap by peers and playmates. Had the families granted these situations fresh, full, and novel recognition (as the research observer was likely to do from his vantage point), they might well have undermined the familiar and binding images of self and other—the sense that it is still the same you and the same I—by which family members had customarily related to one another. This did not happen; but this fact should not be taken to mean, as the families themselves were wont to claim, that, except for a few external facts of life, nothing had changed. On the contrary, there were important changes both in the life situation of the families and in their adjustments to it. But, as we shall also show, such changes were mediated by a variety of psychological masking devices that disguised their experiential contour and gave them the stamp of a familiar and known past.

Clash of Interests Between Hospital and Home

With respect to the often-controversial discussion of family-hospital relations, our findings lead us to reject certain of the more extreme positions taken by critics and commentators in the field. The lesser known of these positions, the functionalist view, conceives of a kind of teleologically fashioned concordance between hospital and home in which each functions beneficially to regulate the primary interests of the other.[14] The more familiar view of the reformers holds not only that present-day hospital practice inflicts serious and sometimes permanent damage on the socio-emotional welfare of the family unit, but also that nearly all such effects could be avoided if only the hospital were made more "homelike" in its atmosphere, routine, and policies.[15] Toward this end a number of changes has been proposed, including unrestricted visiting privileges, rooming-in by parents of hospitalized infants and children, less rigidity in the implementation of various nursing and housekeeping routines, a psychologically more supportive orientation toward patients by staff, and a broadening of the therapeutic focus of medical intervention so as to take into account the influence of family members and other significant persons in the patient's environment.

Of the two views, the former can be dismissed the more readily, despite the elusive appeal of its "whatever is, is right" approach. Just as it can be shown that the hospital relieves the family of certain unmanageable social burdens that illness entails, so it can also be shown that this intervention by the hospital gives rise to other severe burdens that descend upon the family. The problem, then, is as much to assess the respective social costs that the two systems exact from each other as it is to delineate the ways in which they serve each other's purposes. Despite its oversanguine view of the family-hospital relationship, however, the functional approach, with its emphasis on the systemic properties of social structures, does point up certain gaps and doubtful *a priori* assumptions in the reformers' critique. It causes us to be properly skeptical of the degree to which any hospital can, given its distinctive organizational goals and requirements, be made so "homelike" that patients and their families would experience few, if any, disruptions or social imbalances in their lives. If, indeed, the hospital could so modify its organizational character, we might ask whether it would not in the process be subverting some of its legitimate purposes.

[14] Parsons and Fox, *op. cit.*

[15] This view, which has been most strongly stated in certain writings on the effects of hospitalization on children, is closely identified with a group of psychotherapeutically oriented English pediatricians and physicians, particularly Sir James Spence, John Bowlby, and James Robertson. See, for example, James Robertson, *Young Children in Hospitals*, New York: Basic Books, 1958.

These remarks are not intended to gainsay the merit of many of the reformers' proposals. (Even a casual observer cannot but be profoundly struck by the callous, depersonalized, and deadeningly routine treatment meted out in many hospitals nowadays.) One may go even further and grant that the acceptance of these reforms would do much to mitigate the social and psychological stress that hospitalization occasions for families, particularly when the patient is a child. Beyond this, however, we question whether even reforms such as these can produce anything approximating a genuinely harmonious integration of interests and perspectives between the two. Among other reasons, we suggest that in the process of incorporating the hospital's basic therapeutic aims into his motivational system, the patient, especially if he is a child, unavoidably alters and disrupts many of his established ties with his family; further, that in view of this, any radical attempt to shift the treatment emphasis in the direction of the socio-emotional needs of the family threatens to subvert important therapeutic goals. Lastly, we hold that although hospitalization does indeed often result in disruptions and difficulties in family-member relations, the post-confinement severity and duration of these problems bear greater relation to the historic patterning of interpersonal relations in the family than to the hospital experience *per se*.

Stated more generally, the view taken here is that although much can doubtless be done to ameliorate the socially disruptive effects of hospitalization on the family, attempts in this direction are limited by the differences in perspective, goals, and structure of the two systems. Neither can wholly accommodate the other without jeopardizing its own functional integrity as an organization. Hence, major conflicts and strains are bound to arise whenever family and hospital are brought into protracted relations. Much of what follows is addressed to the elucidation of the sources, nature, and consequences of this difficult predicament.

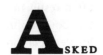

Chapter 2. The Crisis Experience

to describe the onset of his nine-year-old daughter's illness, Mr. Mason,[1] foreman in a lumber mill, gave the following account. He spoke haltingly and quietly, occasionally pausing in his narrative to sniff back tears or clear his throat.

> Well, [Norma Jean] had a little, slight cold that week. . . . But that week, all that week, why, she went to school. We even asked her one morning, I believe, if she wanted to stay home. She said no. . . . She didn't want to lose any time, she said. She didn't seem sick. And Saturday is when we noticed that—you know, she felt worse. But of course she's—Lord, I mean—years previous she's been sicker than that and went to school. We never noticed anything, never given anything like polio a thought. And then Saturday I was working daylight shift and when I came home from work she was out in the lady's yard next door. . . . She said, "Hi, Dad." She acted all right to me, and I didn't even give it a thought about her being sick. Then when she come in, why she started laying around and she acted to me maybe more like

[1] To protect the privacy of the 14 families who participated in the research, pseudonyms are used in this book. Details of occupation and residence, and other facts that might conceivably lead to their identification, have also been disguised. Similarly, doctors, physiotherapists, and other treatment personnel mentioned in these pages are referred to by arbitrarily chosen letter symbols.

she had an upset stomach than she had a cold. . . . And that night . . . I give her a dose of milk of magnesia, just a small dose. And the next morning, why her bowels hadn't moved, and I give her another small dose, and still thinking that it was more of a upset stomach than it was a cold—see, because you could have took it either way. Well, she just laid here on the sofa all day. She watched television. That day some time she started complaining about her leg feeling heavy. And she went upstairs to the bathroom two or three times, without any assistance. I didn't give it a thought, and that Saturday night [the previous evening], though, I told my wife, not giving a thought in the world that anything could happen to us, I said, "You know, I'm always scared about polio." I didn't give it a thought in the world she had it—I'm just thinking, you know. . . . But I didn't think it'd happen to us. And so she laid around all Sunday, and we put a pad on her leg, and I rubbed her leg some. . . . Couple of times I started to rub it, you know, and she told me to stop. And she went to bed, I guess about 9:30 or 10 o'clock, something like that. . . . She ate a good supper and, well, you know, we figured she was eating and all, she was just feeling punk. . . . I told my wife that night, I said, "Well, if she don't feel too good in the morning, call Dr. S." So the next morning she seemed to have a temperature. . . . A little later on her temperature dropped and my wife told her that if her temperature come back again she was going to call Dr. S. And it come back. She called Dr. S. and I don't—I just forget what the temperature was. It was a little high—wasn't even too high, I mean, but it was a little along. And Dr. S. come. She [Norma Jean] didn't want him to come, you know. Now that's one reason my wife was holding off, because she was afraid he was going to give her a needle, see! And my wife was just trying to please her. . . . So after she saw that the temperature did come back . . . she got a little more worried, and then she called Dr. S. and he come, I guess around 2:00 to 3:00, somewhere in around there. I was working. My wife tells me that he closed the bedroom door and come down and started calling right away trying to get an ambulance. He said he—it looked like polio to him. He was going to send her to Eastern Hospital [the receiving center for all polio cases in the area] for sure. Then he called me, and I come home and I rushed her right up to Eastern. . . . Dr. S. called some doctor up there . . . and we took her in the little waiting room there—examination room, I guess you'd call it. This doctor came down in about ten to fifteen minutes. . . . He examined her all over, testing the reflexes and the muscles, you know. So then they put her on a stretcher and took her to the children's ward. And then Dr. R. come in. We was in a waiting room there. He come in and he told us that she definitely had polio. And I was so in doubt, you know, . . . I

said, "Well, ain't you going to take a spinal test? How do you know
she's got it?" He said, "Well, all the symptoms are there." He said,
"We're so sure she's got it that we're not going to put her through that
misery." So then they told us how often we could see her and all, and
how long she'd have to stay there [before being transferred to a convalescent hospital]. We went in to see her, and that was it. And I—
for two or three days after I was still, you know, feeling that, well,
maybe they was wrong. But they wasn't.

Though differing, naturally, in its particulars, Mr. Mason's description of the onset of his daughter's polio encompasses the range and
sequence of events, attitudes, thoughts, and actions that characterized
the unfolding of this crisis[2] in the 14 families studied. Some of the
accounts given by other parents were more dramatic, some were more
commonplace. In some families the events comprising the onset history prior to the critical incident (i.e., the diagnosis of the child's
condition as paralytic poliomyelitis) were only a day or two in duration; in others they were drawn out for almost a week.

Yet, despite the differences in the particularities making up the crisis
histories of the 14 families, the fundamental similarities allow us to
speak of an *essential* or *model* crisis experience. This refers neither
to some dominant statistical patterning of sequential events nor to an
ideal-type configuration of factors, although in itself the concept of an
essential crisis experience need not exclude either of these other con-
structs as analytical alternatives. What I have in mind is the underlying perceptual-interpretative process whereby a family is carried from
a state of relative security and composure regarding its members and
their capacities to a state that it perceives as grossly threatening to
this balance, in part because it challenges the understandings by which
family members customarily relate to one another. Concretely, to see
one's child healthy and active one day and to be forced, a day or so
later, to consider the likelihood of his dying, being crippled, or compelled to live in a mechanical respirator entails a most dramatic and
disruptive alteration in fundamental perspectives.

[2] Perhaps because of the many kinds of crisis situations studied by sociologists, the literature abounds in different definitions of "crisis." I shall use the
term here to designate a relatively sudden and unanticipated disruption, of
extensive and protracted significance, in the everyday activities, understandings,
and expectations of a social unit, in this instance the family.

The perceptual-interpretative process characterizing this shift may be formulated as follows. The parents apply an everyday, minimally threatening explanatory framework (e.g., virus, cold, upset stomach) to their child's apparent illness until certain incongruous perceptions are introduced into the situation (e.g., the child falls, is unable to walk, is febrile for a long period of time). It proves increasingly difficult to rationalize these incongruities within the familiar explanatory framework. The resulting ambiguity casts doubt on the validity of the commonplace explanation. When, or shortly after, they experience such doubts, the parents initiate a course of action (e.g., calling a doctor, rushing the child to a hospital) which eventuates—suddenly in some cases, but in others only after a period of further indecision and vacillation—in a diagnosis of the child's condition as far more serious and dangerous than they had believed at the outset. This medically authoritative diagnosis eventually dispels the parents' first or subsequent explanations of the child's illness, despite the doubts concerning its validity that some of them continue to harbor.

In other words, a commonplace explanatory framework is applied at the onset of the child's illness. With the introduction of incongruous symptoms, this becomes ambiguous and less tenable, giving rise to a course of action that eventuates, sooner or later, in a definition of the child's condition as one more serious and dangerous than that originally contemplated.

THE STAGE ANALYSIS OF CRISIS SITUATIONS

In their attempt to bring some order and meaning to the bewildering complex of events, actions, and feelings that characterizes mass disasters such as floods or tornadoes, social scientists have sought to break down the history of the disasters into sequential stages.[3] These typically include a pre-disaster or quiescent stage, in which the community is seen as going about its normal business; a warning or threat stage, in which signs of the approaching disaster appear but are not always attended to; an impact stage, in which the disaster strikes; a

[3] See D. W. Chapman, ed., "Human Behavior in Disaster: A New Field of Social Research," *Journal of Social Issues*, X, 3 (1954).

post-impact, or inventory, stage, in which the extent of damage and loss is assessed; and, finally, a long-term recovery stage, in which the community attempts to repair the damage and replace its losses.

The advantages of a sequential-stage analysis of this type are obvious. It allows the investigator to break down his subject matter into more manageable parts, to relate these parts to one another in a relatively systematic way, and, in general, to bestow a semblance of analytical order on the chaos of contradictory reports and observations that usually emerges from the disaster experience. In these very advantages, however, lies the chief disadvantage of this approach; for the segmented description of the crisis experience tends to suggest that more order and coherence exist than is usually the case in such situations. To the extent that confusion, vacillation, ambiguity, fortuitousness, and the like distinguish these occurrences from everyday social life—and they clearly do—the employment of this kind of analytical tool falls short of reality. However, neither sociology nor psychology has yet evolved a set of concepts and terminology that more adequately express the suddenness, rapidity, and breadth of social and personal changes experienced in disaster situations.[4]

The analysis of the crisis experience of families that polio strikes poses a not dissimilar dilemma. Here, too, time is stripped of its familiar contexts as new and disturbing events quickly succeed and overlap each other. In most instances, vacillation, foreboding, and uncertainty mark the stance of the participants, as for those in the midst of a mass disaster. Basically, the same paradox of ordering reality versus the unreality of order taunts the investigator who wishes somehow to describe objectively the course of events.

Fully recognizing this dilemma, I shall now attempt to "order" the polio crisis experience in the 14 families according to a set of developmental stages. Following in part the terminology used in mass-disaster studies, I have designated them, in order of their emergence, the

[4] See A. F. C. Wallace, *Human Behavior in Extreme Situations: A Survey of the Literature and Suggestions for Further Research*, Disaster Study No. 1 (National Academy of Sciences, National Research Council, Committee on Disaster Studies, Washington, D.C., 1956), Publication No. 390. Some pertinent observations along these lines are also to be found in A. W. Gouldner, "Theoretical Requirements of the Applied Social Sciences," *American Sociological Review*, XXII (February, 1957), 95.

prelude stage, the warning stage, the impact stage, the inventory stage, and the recovery stage. Since the last of these, recovery, comprises a major focus of this study, it will be discussed in subsequent chapters. Here I shall consider only the first four stages, from prelude through inventory.

THE PRELUDE STAGE

From the standpoint of the family, the prelude stage may be said to extend from the time the parents become aware that the child is "sick," or "not feeling well" to the time they apprehend some cue that his indisposition might not be of the "ordinary" kind. Until such cues were perceived, almost all the families studied thought that the child was suffering from a cold, stomach upset, "virus," overfatigue, or some other common childhood ailment. These diagnostic inferences followed quite naturally in most instances from the child's beginning complaint—a sore throat, stomach ache, feeling of tiredness, headache, or some combination of these. The concomitant incidence of nausea, constipation, listlessness, or slight fever appeared to support the parents' initial diagnosis, and in virtually all cases they administered such antidotes as aspirin, a laxative, an enema, a tonic, or some other simple home remedy. Some parents immediately sent the child to bed, some called the family doctor, others restricted the child's play or diet, and a few did nothing at all, assuming that the ailment was minor and would pass in short order.

Whatever the specific therapeutic path followed by the parents, the remedial measures they adopted at this early point in the crisis history were for the most part simple, commonsensical, and in accord with popular (and by no means medically disparaged) practice in dealing with a child who has a slight cold or is feeling "run down," tired, or "out of sorts."[5]

[5] The absence of quack remedies or outlandish forms of treatment among all these families was striking, particularly in view of their class composition. This may, of course, have been due to the familiarity of the ailments that the children were thought to have at first. Even so, this finding would seem to challenge to some degree the oft-repeated view that large numbers of families in our society, particularly those of lower socioeconomic status, automatically resort to grossly inappropriate and even harmful "remedies" when illness strikes.

At this early stage, however, many parents (seven of the fourteen) would not even wholly admit that the child was ill. In four of these families the sick child had previously been involved in some incident or mishap that might have accounted for his complaints; hence, the usual definition of the beginning illness as a cold, sore throat, or stomach upset was not applied in these cases. For example, several days before he began complaining of feeling ill, six-year-old Neil Richards had been in a schoolyard tussle with a classmate who reportedly jumped on Neil's back. Mrs. Richards, in describing the onset of Neil's illness, stated: "He said he didn't feel good. He had a stomach ache. . . . And he told me at school some little boy had jumped on his back and his back was hurting him and I thought then that it was just from that." (Interpretations of this kind, it might be noted, often persisted in attenuated form after other ones suggested themselves, sometimes even after the doctor had rendered a diagnosis of paralytic polio.)

In three other families, the parents questioned the legitimacy of the child's complaints in the belief that he might be feigning illness so as to win attention and indulgence.[6] According to Mrs. Baker, for example, when her son Gerald complained of a stiff neck, "I thought he was just playing, because sometimes when he's sick he loves to be pampered, you know. And he likes his meals brought up to bed to him." None of these families entertained this particular misconstruction of the child's onset illness for long. In effect they tested the possibility that the child was malingering (as, apparently, all three children in question were known to have done before), found this hypothesis inadequate, and then quickly dropped it in favor of some other explanation.

Not only those parents who at first thought that the child's complaint of illness was psychologically motivated but also, to a somewhat

[6] It is interesting to note that in each of these families the child suspected of feigning illness was not only the oldest sibling but male as well. (In two of the families he was the elder of two children, and in the third the oldest of five.) The question naturally arises whether this expectation is characteristically associated with the status of oldest male sibling, and, if so, why? It may have some thing to do with the greater responsibility usually assigned the oldest male child in the family. This may predispose him to resort to the sick role as a legitimate means of relinquishing responsibility; at the same time, it may cause the parents to be extrasensitive to the possibility of his doing so. See T. Parsons and R. Fox, "Illness, Therapy and the Modern Urban American Family," *Journal of Social Issues,* VIII, 4 (1952), 31-44.

lesser extent, those who believed that the symptoms were the result of a mishap seemed to have difficulty in defining their child's condition as "illness" in the usual sense. In their view, only organically generated conditions—such as colds, nausea, and, of course, polio—warranted this designation. On reflection, this attitude appears to be connected with the highly ambivalent view popularly taken toward volitional elements in illness. The more it appears that a pathological state is "brought on" through the willful action or carelessness of the individual, the more likely it is that the condition will be defined as a moral or behavioral deviation of some kind rather than as an illness.[7]

The tendency to attribute volitional elements to the illness was strikingly revealed in interviews with the polio children themselves, particularly the younger ones, shortly after their admission to the receiving hospital. Not knowing yet that they had polio—or, if they did, not knowing quite what this meant—they frequently gave as the cause of their paralysis "running around too much," "playing when my mother said I shouldn't," or "falling down when I played too rough." In other words, the paralysis was seen as a kind of punishment for a behavorial transgression.

On a more sophisticated level, the parents showed similar tendencies as they sought to reassure themselves that nothing within their control had been responsible for the child's contracting the disease. Several of them, for example, after having told the interviewer that they could not think of anything that might have accounted for the child's polio, would ask him in an "offhand" manner whether polio was ever caused by eating pork, or playing with a cat or a parakeet, or living in an area where freshly dug earth was being moved for highway or building construction.

For all the families, though, one of the most sinister aspects of the experience in retrospect was the degree to which the early symptoms resembled those of a cold, stomach upset, or other everyday ailment. Doctors themselves are frequently deceived by the first symptoms of

[7] For an excellent discussion of the social norms governing the sick role in our society, see Parsons and Fox, *ibid.* Society's predication of a volitional element in much illness is, of course, even more striking in the case of persons who are eventually diagnosed as mentally ill. See M. R. Yarrow, *et al.,* "The Psychological Meaning of Mental Illness," *Journal of Social Issues,* XI, 4 (1955), 22-23.

polio, and it is only when signs of paralysis appear that the average practitioner will cautiously venture a diagnosis of polio.[8] It is not surprising, therefore, that several of the parents, completely stunned by the final diagnosis, questioned its validity at first, pointing out to the doctor that the child did not seem to be very sick or "that bad off." In retrospect, the deceptively commonplace appearance of the pro-dromal symptoms imparted elements of unreality, even treachery, to the whole crisis experience.

THE WARNING STAGE

The warning stage may be said to begin when the parents perceive some cue suggesting that the child's illness is not simple or ordinary but is perhaps of a more serious nature. Although in most cases such cues specifically suggested polio to the parents, two families began to fear rheumatic fever, and a third thought the child might have a severely injured ankle. What is significant, however, is that the intro-duction of such cues placed a strain on the parents' earlier, common-sensical diagnosis of the child's illness, and ultimately made it wholly untenable. These cues, then, may also be thought of as marking the terminal point of the prelude stage.

Great variability was shown, among and within families, in the time at which the cue was perceived, its sources, and the response made to it. Basic to a consideration of warning cues is the question of the family's prior knowledge of the symptoms, course, and possible outcome of polio. Unfortunately, although all parents were inter-viewed within a week following the child's admission to the hospital, it was not possible to determine with certainty how much they knew prior to the diagnosis and how much they had learned subsequently. In swiftly developing and tremendously disorienting crisis situations of this type, it is exceedingly difficult even for the participants, much more for the researcher, to accurately disentangle prior and subse-quent knowledge. What follows, therefore, is based more on the

[8] In two families where the parents did suspect polio and called a doctor very soon after the child began to complain of feeling ill, the doctor assured them that the cause was not polio but summer grippe or some other inconse-quential virus infection.

interviewer's impressions than on the actual verbal content of the interviews.

The over-all impression is that, with the exception of the Ellsworth family,[9] the parents in the study knew little about polio. In nearly all the families, one or both parents knew of someone—a distant friend, a neighbor, a co-worker—who had had polio or whose child had had polio—and this, apparently, had made them aware of the possibly crippling effects of the disease. However, they could relate very little else regarding its outcomes. All but one or two of the parents knew that a stiff neck was a common symptom of polio, but hardly any knew of any of the other onset symptoms. (Since a stiff neck is by no means always associated with the onset of the disease, this isolated bit of information proved of little value to them.) Mainly because of the Salk-vaccine publicity at the time, almost all the parents were vaguely aware that the disease was somehow caused by a virus, but they were ignorant of the neuro-physiological action of the virus— even as a layman might depict it.[10]

At least one spouse in seven of the families seemed to know that not all poliomyelitis was of the paralytic variety and that paralysis did not inevitably follow infection by the virus. But, despite this information, the popular polio imagery of iron lung, crippling, and death proved too potent to afford them much consolation once they realized that their child had contracted the disease.

Save for the Ellsworths, therefore, the families did not differ greatly in their relatively meager knowledge of the disease before its onset. Such small differences as could be reliably detected among them proved, as we shall see, to be of only minor significance in the subsequent unfolding of the crisis history.

Timing of the Cue

The point in the crisis history at which warning cues were perceived varied considerably from family to family. In some, the cues were detected within a few hours after the child complained of feeling ill;

[9] In this family, both husband and wife had attended college. Further, the husband had worked during World War II in military hospitals, where he came into contact with servicemen being treated for paralytic polio.

[10] The pathology of spinal poliomyelitis is described in Chap. 3, pp. 48-51.

in others, this was delayed almost until the child's admission to the receiving hospital. Most parents, however, were led to question, though not necessarily to revise, their initial view of the child's ailment only after he had been ill for a day or two and then suddenly showed symptoms or behavior for which they could not easily account. We can infer, therefore, that the time at which the warning cue was perceived was largely a function of the rapidity with which the disease progressed during the onset phase—itself a variable matter. For most of the parents, it was not until the development of paralysis—the first clear and dramatic sign of the disease—that the warning stage commenced.

Source of the Cue

The sources of the warning cue may be classified as symptomatological, behavioral, environmental, or authoritative. By symptomatological cues we mean those emanating from the child's physical condition as such—for example, falling down suddenly, being unable to stand, or dragging a leg. Behavioral cues are those perceived as a result of some striking discrepancy in the child's everyday behavior. Mr. Baker, for example, reported that when he saw his three-year-old son, Jim, gain the upper hand in a living-room tussle with six-year-old Gerald he knew that there was something very wrong with the older boy. Environmental cues are those that derive from the time-place context of the child's illness. The Mannings, for example, considered the possibility of polio almost from the start of their daughter's illness because several cases had recently been reported in their neighborhood. Other parents mentioned that polio crossed their minds whenever their children became ill during the summer or early fall months. Authoritative cues are those communicated by a doctor, either openly or through indirection. In three families, for example, a doctor was called in to examine the child more as a precautionary measure than in response to some clear warning perceived by the family. Dr. G., following his examination of five-year-old David Prince, is reported to have told the mother, "I'll be frank with you, Mrs. Prince. The child has either summer grippe or polio. It's too soon to tell—the symptoms are so much alike. We'll have to keep a close watch on him." In the Richards family, polio was never mentioned during the doctor's first visit, but the mother was cued in when she saw the doctor testing for signs of neck stiffness and recalled that this was one of the signs of polio.

Although warning cues of the symptomatological type were the first to be perceived by most parents, it was rare for cues to emanate from one source alone. Typically, the perception of one cue triggered off others, which then fed into each other to produce pronounced strain on the "normal outlook" with which the child's illness had been viewed.

Response to the Cue

The first warning cues elicited different reactions, not only from family to family and parent to parent but even from the same individual as his original definition of the child's condition grew less tenable. For general descriptive purposes, the multivarious reactions can be reduced to three main types: rationalization, reinterpretation, and vacillation.

Some parents attempted somehow to assimilate the warning cue to the commonsensical diagnosis of the child's illness that they had held from the first. Thus, when they first became aware of muscular weakness or rigidity in some part of the child's body, they assumed that the cold had "settled" in the legs, abdomen, or feet, as the case might be.[11] A strong denial component was frequently subsumed by the rationalization response. For example, although Mrs. Lawson claimed to have

[11] The conception of an illness moving through the body and "settling," almost arbitrarily, in one or several parts is interesting in itself and might be termed the "layman's migratory theory of pathology." As a simplification of such technically sophisticated medical designations as residual inflammation and referred pain—phenomena that some laymen might have difficulty grasping and that many practitioners are averse to explain in the belief that they cannot be grasped by laymen—the migratory theory seems to provide a ready-made rule-of-thumb explanation for a host of transient somatic and psychosomatic pains. These are usually of a kind that experience teaches us are too vague to take seriously or to see a doctor about. It would be interesting to determine the relative extent to which this popular concept of pathological process derives from modern, greatly popularized developments in virology or from more primitive etiological notions (e.g., spreading poisons in the body, the entrance of evil spirits, and the ingestion of symbolically evil substances). The ideational affinity of certain modern concepts of disease with more primitive notions is discussed by J. Z. Bowers, "Today's Medicine in Underdeveloped Areas," *Journal of the American Medical Association,* CLIII (November 28, 1953), 1167-71.

thought at once of polio on previous occasions when her children became ill, her awareness seemed to have deserted her at this crucial time: "I didn't bother too much when he said his legs hurt him, because I thought that was just his weak spot, and when he gets grippe or virus like that, it probably hurts him there." The tendency to rationalize was especially marked among parents who interpreted the child's illness in the light of some prior mishap. The injury that had been received, actually or allegedly, afforded a ready-made point of reference for explaining away the pains and soreness of which the child complained.

With the sole exception of the Ellsworths, none of the parents exhibited a clear-cut reinterpretative response to the warning cue (i.e., a decisive revision of their earlier diagnosis of the child's illness). This apparently was true not only because of the parents' understandable reluctance to fix on something so threatening as polio, but also because the child's symptoms were so ambiguous that, for a while at least, the earlier explanation continued to seem at least somewhat plausible.

For the large majority of families, however, the warning cues initiated a period of vacillation that persisted until the child was assigned a bed in the receiving hospital. This was particularly true of parents who had thought of polio but were inclined to dismiss its possibility as too farfetched. (Even when the child was hospitalized, some parents continued to express doubt whether their child "really had polio.") At this stage of the crisis history the parents typically fluctuated in their thinking between "Oh, it's just a cold" and "Maybe it *is* polio." Optimism and pessimism succeeded each other with great rapidity as the child's condition fluctuated between quiescence and activity. Recurring visions of disaster were cushioned by an indulgent self-chastisement in which the parent told himself that he "gets alarmed too easily." For example, the mother of seven-year-old Edward Short reported:

Well, I'll tell you the truth. We didn't—we might have thought of polio, but we didn't want to. We just didn't want to think of it I guess, even though he wouldn't walk. . . . But that night I said to my husband when he was getting ready to take him to the doctor, I said, "I can't hardly believe that he could possibly have polio." I said, "Look, I can move his legs." And I went to move one and he yelled out, and that almost knocked me over. I just stood there, almost—just—I just didn't know what to say. So I thought then, "Well, I bet it is." But I didn't want to think about it.

Of interest in this connection is the manner in which the meaning of the warning cue was communicated between family members. In certain families, one parent suspected polio but said nothing lest he alarm his spouse unduly; nevertheless, according to their accounts, each knew what was on the other's mind. According to Mr. Ellsworth, for example, his wife learned that he suspected polio when she observed him examining their daughter's neck for signs of stiffness. In this family the hidden dialogue was extended to include the family doctor as well. Mrs. Ellsworth told how Dr. B., by directing her attention to the reflex tests he performed during his first examination of Sarah, enabled her to "discuss" with him the possibility of polio without ever mentioning the word.

In those families in which the parents discussed the possibility of polio, it was usual for one of them—generally the father, although not always—to assume the role of comforter, attempting to reassure his mate that "it probably isn't polio at all" but something much less serious. Needless to say, a parent often assumed the role of mate comforter despite his own grave doubts. Perhaps because the mate-comforting role had been performed too assiduously at first, a role reversal occurred in at least two of the families, the comforter becoming the comforted once the child's illness was definitely diagnosed as paralytic polio. It was as if the parent had been so strongly committed to the emotional content of the role that he could not reassume it once he had been proved wrong. For example, when Mrs. Harris voiced her fears to her husband, two days prior to her son's diagnosis as a polio case, Mr. Harris assured her, and continued to do so until he took the boy to the doctor, that Marvin's leg pains were only the aftereffects of a roller-skating fall some two weeks earlier. Upon the child's admission to the receiving hospital Mr. Harris "went to pieces," and it became necessary for Mrs. Harris to assume the role of comforter toward him.

This digression into questions of family interaction touches on matters to be considered in detail elsewhere. Here I want only to point out that the kind and degree of the parents' response to warning cues, once perceived, varied with role relationships in the family, the progress of the disease itself, and sheer fortuitous circumstance. Clearly, what we see are reactions built up according to some emergent pattern rather than simply elicited by stimuli.

THE IMPACT STAGE

For the majority of families, what we have termed the warning stage overlapped the impact stage: that period, generally of short duration, in which the family learned that the child's illness was in fact paralytic poliomyelitis and came, more or less, to accept the diagnosis. Differences from family to family in the degree to which these two stages overlapped stemmed, as I have suggested, from variations in the nature and intensity of the warning cues, in the timing of their perception by the parents, and in the parents' responses to these cues. For some, the definitive medical diagnosis of paralytic poliomyelitis represented an inexorable fulfillment of their worst fears. For others, it came as a startling, almost ironic, recognition that what had crossed their minds and had been too readily dismissed as "farfetched" or "improbable" had indeed come to pass. For still others, it was a shattering rebuke to carefully cultivated reasonableness to discover that it was not, after all, the roller-skating fall or playground tussle that accounted for their child's illness.

Even some of those families who had considered the possibility of polio actively resisted the diagnosis at first, voicing such doubts as "Maybe the doctors are wrong," "How can they tell without taking a spinal tap?" and "If another doctor examined him he would find out that it's not polio at all." Only the passage of time and the exacerbation of the early paralytic symptoms appeared to convince these parents of the correctness of the doctor's diagnosis.

Of considerable relevance in this connection were the diagnostic actions and communications of the family doctor. In eight of the families only one visit by the family doctor preceded the child's hospitalization. At this visit the doctor made a tentative diagnosis of polio or of some broadly related disease (e.g., meningitis unspecified, spinal meningitis). In those families in which the doctor made several visits, he may have hinted at the possibility of polio, but almost always hedged to some degree in his final pre-hospitalization diagnosis. In several cases the doctor conveyed his suspicions by mentioning not polio specifically but some condition similar to it of which the parents generally knew less, though perhaps enough to take the hint. Some of the family doctors pronounced no diagnosis at all at this time, but urged the parents to take the child immediately to Eastern Hospital, where, they told the parents, "they have the set-up to make the tests that will tell us what's wrong." This hospital was the sole receiving center for polio cases in the area, a fact of which the doctors were certainly aware but of which the families were not. Most of the doctors did go so far as to state that they thought the child had polio, usually adding, however, that this could not be definitely determined until the child was examined at Eastern Hospital.

Certain aspects of the interaction between the parents and the family doctor during the impact stage deserve comment. We might note, at the outset, that the doctors' unwillingness to make a firm diagnosis of polio seemed to serve several purposes simultaneously, some better than others. First, it afforded the doctors some protection in the event that their tentative diagnosis was proved wrong. It was not very likely to be discredited, especially where the child already showed definite signs of paralysis, as nearly all of them did at this point. But in view of its conceivably great bearing on the doctor's future relationship with the family, not to mention his professional reputation, it is understandable why the physician in his role of family doctor would be motivated to take this precaution.

Secondly, it relieved the doctor to some extent of the unpleasant task of "breaking the bad news" to the parents. The responsibility for this bit of "dirty work"[12] passed largely to the more impersonal, less involved medical authorities at the receiving hospital (residents, internes), who were more or less shielded by their organizational cloak against the recriminations sometimes directed at physicians in cases of severe illness.

Finally, the doctors' tendency to hedge the pre-hospitalization diagnosis stemmed from their wish to believe that the family would prove better able to face up to the ensuing crisis if the unwelcome diagnosis was divulged bit by bit rather than all at once. More often than not, however, the parents, in their eagerness to have their fears dispelled, took the doctor's diagnostic qualifications too literally. Thus, they

[12] I am indebted to Everett C. Hughes for pointing out the relevance of the concept of "dirty work" for certain facets of medical practice.

persisted in the hope that he would be proved wrong once the child was "thoroughly examined" at the receiving hospital. The Masons, for example, protested the hospital doctors' verdict of polio because no spinal puncture had been made on their daughter, Norma Jean. They had been told by their family doctor that this would be done in order "to make sure." Similarly, several days after her son's admission to Eastern Hospital, Mrs. Lawson expressed to the interviewer doubt whether John really had polio. She had been told by her family doctor that a spinal tap was the only sure test for polio, and none had been made on John.[13]

As we shall see in Chapter 3, the pre-hospitalization interaction between parents and family doctor, with its veiled hints, qualifications, and equivocality, served in many ways as a model for the family's subsequent contacts with persons responsible for the child's treatment and care. In effect, it marked the initiation of the family into a world in which as much is left unsaid as is said, and in which the art of "hearing between the lines" comes disturbingly into its own.

To return to the chronological account of events at this stage, there was surprisingly little variation from family to family in the impact experiences as a whole. Although the families had followed somewhat different paths in reaching this point in the crisis history, once the child was hospitalized, the institutionalized regularities of hospital practice provided the parents with a relatively common frame of reference. Following the family doctor's instructions, the parents took the child to Eastern Hospital, where they usually waited for several hours while the child was examined, a medical history was taken, and, in some cases, a spinal tap was made. The attending physicians as a rule declined to comment about the child's condition until all the diagnostic findings were in. This tended to increase the anxious suspense of the parents' vigil. Finally, confirmation of the family doctor's tentative diagnosis was brought in, and the parents were told that they would have to leave the child at the hospital. Beyond this, they were told little about his condition at this time.

This point may be regarded as the high-water mark of the crisis

---

[13] Hospital physicians are reluctant to administer the spinal-tap test because it causes the child sharp pain. In the more obvious cases of paralytic involvement, where there is little need for additional evidence of polio, doctors frequently dispense with the test in order to spare the child discomfort.

history. In its immediate wake followed a number of developments of long-range social-psychological significance, not least of which was, of course, the separation of child and parents. In view of the extended discussion of these developments in later chapters, I shall deal here only with matters of particular relevance to the impact stage as such. Chief among these are the immediate emotional reactions of the parents to the diagnosis of paralytic polio and the imagery that it called forth. Most described extreme feelings of helplessness and personal loss. Weeping was a common reaction to the diagnosis.

Personally, I cried. We cried all night long. [Mr. Short]

I just couldn't hold up. . . . I don't ever remember crying so hard. My eyes were covered with sties from so much crying. [Mrs. Prince]

When I heard them say polio it was like someone was pulling my heart out. [Mr. Baker]

In most of the families, the fathers as well as the mothers reportedly wept and "broke down" upon hearing the diagnosis. In retrospect, the fathers themselves tended to describe this reaction as simply a temporary loss of control. This fissure in "normal" masculine behavior may have helped foster a stronger sense of family solidarity, a development that many parents later identified as a positive by-product of the crisis experience. Conventionally interpreted, weeping by men in our society connotes an extraordinary degree of affective involvement. This demonstration dramatically reassured the wives of an identity of interest and sentiment between spouses that is sometimes left open to question in routine, fairly uneventful, family life.[14]

Underlying the profound emotional reactions of the parents was the imagery of crippling, iron lungs, and death that the polio diagnosis triggered. Mr. Richards remarked, "Well, we worried about whether he would ever walk again, or be in one of those iron lungs or in a wheelchair, whether he would be crippled bad or have to wear built-up shoes." The little girl in braces on the March of Dimes poster and

[14] Similar solidarity reactions have frequently been noted among the victims of mass disasters. Cf. Charles E. Fritz, "Disaster," in R. K. Merton and R. A. Nisbet, eds., *Contemporary Social Problems*, New York: Harcourt, Brace, and World, 1961, pp. 682-92.

the newsreel shots of the wedding of the man in the iron lung some-times flashed across the parent's mind. In several families the parents suddenly remembered having heard about "a man at work" or "a lady in the neighborhood" whose little boy or girl had died of polio. Vivid personal memories of crippled friends and acquaintances frequently intruded themselves on the parent's consciousness.

Extreme and demoralizing as such imagery was, we shall see that its occurrence came to serve as an important reference point for the family in their subsequent conceptions of the child's condition and prospects for recovery.

THE INVENTORY STAGE

The inventory stage is the period, usually within a day or two after the impact experience, in which the families attempt to assess what has happened and to try "to make some sense of it." Even more than the preceding stages, this stage is difficult to delimit precisely in time. For a few families, especially those who had had early suspicions of polio, this stage coincided with or even preceded the impact experience. The atypical Ellsworths, for example, having strongly suspected for several days prior to their daughter's hospitalization that she had con-tracted polio, began at this pre-impact point to wonder how serious her involvement would be. For two families at the other extreme, the inventory stage was delayed because of the parents' inability to calm down sufficiently to reflect on what had happened. When, for exam-ple, four-year-old Frankie Lee was admitted to Eastern Hospital, Mrs. Lee was reduced to a near-hysterical state of grief. She ran off to her mother's house for several days while her husband and older son managed for themselves at home as best they could. During this period she was unable to compose herself sufficiently to take stock.

During the inventory stage, many life concerns, in addition to the physical condition of the child, were brought up for review. These ranged from the most eschatological (e.g., "What was God's purpose in singling out our child for so dreadful a disease?") to the most mundane (e.g., installing a phone in the home so that the parents would not have to bother neighbors when they wanted to call the hospital). All these matters had some relevance for the crisis experience and the long recovery period that followed, but here we shall confine our discussion to the parents' evaluation of the child's condition, their feelings of responsibility for it, and the meaning with which they imbued the crisis experience, particularly as this last affected their sense of relatedness to the scheme of everyday life with which they were familiar.

Evaluation of the Child's Condition

The demoralizing imagery accompanying the diagnosis was very soon counterbalanced by second thoughts of a more optimistic nature. Even those parents who sought temporary refuge in questioning the diagnosis soon accepted its validity for all practical purposes and began to develop rudimentary anticipatory strategies for estimating the child's injury and prospects for recovery. These early optimistic re-appraisals were usually expressed in such terms as "It's not so bad as we thought at first," "He's got the will power to lick the thing," or quite simply, "We believe that he'll come out of it all right."

Among the many factors in the immediate post-impact situation that contributed to this re-evaluation, perhaps the foremost was the parents' early realization that the child was going to survive and was not going to spend his life in an iron lung dwelling on the borderline of death. The location of the paralysis in the lower extremities usually permitted the receiving-hospital doctors to extend this minimum reassurance, at least, to the parents. In light of their previous knowledge that some paralytic-polio victims do go into mechanical respirators and that some of them do die of the disease, such reassurance relieved the parents to a considerable extent of the dire expectations first occasioned by the diagnosis.[15] As one mother, Mrs. Lawson, put it:

> When you think of polio you think of those people in respirators and not being able to move at all. . . . I'm thankful it's just his leg. Of

[15] This phenomenon has been termed "relative deprivation" by R. K. Merton and A. S. Kitt. Relative to parents of healthy children (a positive reference group), the polio parents felt deprived; relative to parents of iron-lung victims or of children who had died (a negative reference group), they thought themselves fortunate. See R. K. Merton and P. F. Lazarsfeld, *Studies on the Scope and Method of "The American Soldier,"* Glencoe, Ill.: Free Press, 1950, pp. 42-53.

course it's a terrible thing for a child not to be able to walk or not to be entirely like other children, but at least he's here, and I always think it could be worse.

Secondly, once the gross threats of respiratory involvement and imminent death were ruled out, the medical indefiniteness and apparent uncertainty of the situation, particularly when viewed against the backdrop of the optimistic bias of American mores, allowed the parents no psychologically viable alternative other than hope for a total, or near-total, recovery. (At this stage the doctors refused to prognosticate on the ultimate extent of the child's paralytic involvement or on his chances for muscle recovery.) To the extent that the parents felt impelled to develop some working concept of the future, they tended to shape it along highly favorable lines. One father, Mr. Short, expressed this anticipatory dilemma rather explicitly. Asked what went through his mind when he first learned that his son had polio, he replied:

> Well, I suppose the fear that the boy would be crippled for life, or perhaps in a wheelchair. I mean, you don't want to think about those things because you want to shove them back as far as you can, even though you know he has polio. I think my son can lick it now, because I want to believe that. If I believe otherwise—well, I'm licked myself. If you don't think that you have nothing to look forward to really.

Finally, the families' great implicit faith and trust in the restorative powers of modern medicine buttressed their relatively optimistic reappraisals of the situation. This attitude, so basic in the life scheme of the contemporary American family, was brought preformed, so to speak, to the situation. Apparently it required only the ruling out of extreme contingencies to become operative.

It would be incorrect, however, to conclude that the optimistic reevaluations of the inventory stage were so pervasive as to exclude less favorable outlooks. Nor did this optimistic frame of mind persist throughout the months of the child's hospitalization. Rather, it was as if a fluctuating internal dialectic was generated, in which the despair of the impact stage and the hopefulness of the inventory stage constantly modified and sought to come to terms with each other.

Parents' Evaluation of Their Own Responsibility

Although the very nature of polio does not, medically speaking, permit one to speak of "responsibility" for a child's contracting the disease,[16] questions in this area loomed large in the family's thoughts. The relatively sudden, unanticipated paralysis of the child appeared to challenge in a number of fundamental respects the parents' conceptions of themselves as responsible and devoted mothers and fathers. It also led them to wonder whether the sick child himself might have committed certain transgressions that led to his contracting the disease and for which they, as parents, were ultimately responsible.[17] Mr. Richards, for example, said of his wife: "I reckon she was so upset because she had the idea maybe she could have done something to keep him from getting it." Mr. Mason said: "It's been running through my mind where could she've gotten it, or what has she done wrong to get it. I can't figure it. It's too deep for me."

The concern over one's own responsibility for the crisis would seem to be associated with still another key assumption in the American value scheme: namely, that misfortune rarely touches those who take the proper precautionary measures. This essentially pragmatic outlook conditions everyday thought and action even in spheres that still lie outside the realm of rational-scientific control. (This may be an instance of cultural pacing, as distinguished from cultural lag; that is, principles of scientific control operative in the technological sphere come to be so widely assimilated in popular thought that they are then mechanically and inappropriately applied to problems that are less amenable to narrowly technical solution.)[18] As regards polio, for example, there is little evidence to suggest that a person's activities

[16] It will be recalled that the study was carried out during the two years immediately prior to the mass introduction of the Salk vaccine program. Hence, there was nothing the parents could have done to prevent their children from contracting the disease.

[17] As noted earlier, it was the children themselves, particularly the younger ones, who tended to give overt expression to this retributive type of causal thinking.

[18] The classic treatment of what I have called cultural pacing with reference to matters of economic and political organization is Karl Mannheim, *Man and Society in an Age of Reconstruction*, New York: Harcourt, Brace, 1944, pp. 51-65. On cultural lag, see W. F. Ogburn, *Social Change*, New York: Viking, 1922.

can be so controlled as to eliminate exposure to the various strains of the virus. Yet for years, until the development of the Salk vaccine, parents were sternly cautioned to keep their children away from crowds, public swimming places, and the like during the summer and early fall months. It is not surprising, therefore, that the parents worried about what they might have done wrong—whether the trip to the amusement park or the public beach had been wise, or whether they should have been more careful in supervising the child's play habits.

Even had they not disregarded such dubious warnings, the parents might still have blamed themselves, for the practical, insurance-minded American attitude toward misfortune can in itself give rise to guilt feelings of a theological or metaphysical kind.[19] Here the belief is that the family is somehow guilty of having pursued a faulty scheme of life that in unknown but predetermined ways resulted in misfortune to the child. Mr. Baker gave eloquent expression to this type of thinking:

> I think it's just an inner-self letdown that you as a parent have not guided your family and your household the way that you would have guided it had you known this was coming. Let's put it this way. Suppose instead of living here, suppose a month ago I was living in the state of Washington. Why didn't I decide to go to the state of Washington instead of living here? . . . What made me come here? I don't know. No one else knows. But I did, I did come here. Here's where Gerry got sick. Here's where he contracted the disease. Is that my fault? I was calling the tricks. Why didn't I pick them somewhere else? I played the wrong card. I got caught. It was my fault. That's what goes through your mind. That's what you think. Your better judgment says, we can't control these things. We know we can't. But it's still there. It's still something to think about.

In other families the belief, or feeling, that the child's disease was retribution for unknown transgressions was expressed in more conventional ways such as, "What have we done that God has singled us out for this?"[20] At this level, some of the parents took the resigned

[19] Cf. Renée C. Fox, *Experiment Perilous*. Glencoe, Ill.: Free Press, 1959, pp. 132-35.

[20] An interesting discussion of the role of retributive themes in the causal thinking of primitive and modern peoples is to be found in H. Kelsen, *Society and Nature*, Chicago: University of Chicago Press, 1947.

view that the child's paralysis was the result of divine will. One Catholic family, for example, chose to regard it as a stigma indicative of their son's blessedness and calling to the cloth.

It is doubtful whether the parents ever completely resolved their conjectures about their responsibility for the child's illness. For the most part, however, such guilt as they felt was soon assuaged, in a number of characteristic ways. A primary source of absolution was the doctor's assurance that there was nothing the parents could have done to lessen the severity of the child's illness, much less to prevent his contracting it in the first place. For more than half the families, prayer and consultation with a minister or priest helped to relieve the conscience of the parents. Several of them claimed to have moved "closer to God" as a result of the crisis. Judging from later interviews, this renewed religious impulse did not always persist with undiminished vigor. It should be noted, however, that the devotional state forms so conspicuous a part of the conventional image of the good, caring parent that its assumption at this time undoubtedly helped the parents to re-establish this identity for themselves.

Perhaps the most effective source of reassurance to the family of its blamelessness was the support and sympathy extended to it by the community. After some initial hesitation due to fear of contagion, neighbors and relatives rallied around the family; they inquired after the sick child, expressed condolences, helped with baby-sitting and other household-management problems, sent the child cards and presents, and in some instances even made offers of financial assistance to the family. Co-workers of the husband demonstrated similar concern and compassion. Classmates of the sick child composed reports for him in which each individually wished him a speedy recovery. Special prayers were said for the family at church. Slight acquaintances— even strangers—visited or telephoned to wish the family well. Encouraging reports flowed in from friends and neighbors of other children who had had polio and "came out of it without a mark." What might otherwise have proved a crushing financial burden for the family was relieved almost immediately—for some by Blue Cross initially, but in the long run for all by the sizable and virtually unconditional aid extended by the local chapter of the National Foundation for Infantile Paralysis.[21]

Clearly, these were not the reactions or sentiments that genuinely and manifestly "guilty" parents would have elicited from their community. Although it was probably not intended for this purpose, the barrage of attention and sympathy from friends and neighbors clearly played an important part in mitigating the parents' feelings that they might have been negligent or were otherwise blameworthy for the child's illness.

Evaluation of the Meaning of the Crisis

Guilt, warranted or not, was but one facet of the threat the disease posed to the values and identities of the family members. Paralytic polio, as the parents were only too well aware, might mean crippling, and to be crippled or to have someone in one's family who is crippled is not, in the parents' words, "the normal thing." In our society, crippling not only signifies a relative loss of physical mobility but also suggests social abnormality, isolation, and, in the eyes of some, visible manifestation of inherent malevolence.[22] The effects of this threat on the family's conception of itself and its relationship to "normal" families (or some idealized image of the normal family) were considerable. The part it played during the whole course of the child's illness and

[21] Reversing the usual welfare pattern, the local branch of the National Foundation for Infantile Paralysis sought out the families upon being notified of polio admissions by the hospital. Only the most brief and general questions were asked concerning each family's financial position. Repayment not being expected, nothing was said about it, although many parents voluntarily promised to make repayment, in part at least. Interestingly, a few of the parents in the study held the view that the financial aid extended them by the Foundation was a form of insurance payment, a return on their contributions over the years to the March of Dimes and other Foundation fund-raising drives. Some of the doctors questioned expressed strong resentment against the Foundation for what they regarded as overindulgent policies toward polio families. They felt that such subsidies not only were an ominous precursor of socialized medicine but also engendered lax and unappreciative attitudes in the families toward the medical care and treatment that the child received.

[22] For a cross-cultural comparison of the status of the crippled and handicapped, see R. G. Barker *et al., Adjustment to Physical Handicap and Illness: A Survey of the Social Psychology of Physique and Disability,* New York: SSRC Bulletin 55, Revised 1953.

recovery will be dealt with in a later chapter. Here I wish only to call attention to some of its beginning manifestations.

Of central importance, though rarely expressed overtly by the parents, was the apparent feeling that the family was no longer "like everyone else." Despite—or perhaps because of—the reassurance, support, and sympathy of the community, the parents felt that others regarded them, and they regarded themselves, as a family upon whom misfortune had been visited. Although misfortune is no doubt distributed throughout the general population, it is a truism that the American image of the good life is predicated on the proposition that calamity may befall others but will not touch one's immediate family. Almost without exception, the parents reflected on this aspect of the crisis experience. Mr. Short, for example, commented:

> You wonder about it. You can't believe it's happened to you. You think, well, it's maybe so many cases in the United States every year, but it's never here. It's always next door, or next county, or next state. Never here. It has to hit somewhere sometime, but you never think of yourself. And this time it was us.

We may surmise, therefore, that the shocking contradiction of the "it can't happen to us" hypothesis severely taxed the family's sense of sharing in a common universe of "normal" experience. This shift in the family's self-image, from a group more or less like other families, with a "normal" quota of satisfactions and troubles, to one that had been "singled out" for misfortune, constituted one of the most alienative features of the crisis experience. Although the parents were barely conscious of this change and did not articulate it in these terms, it nevertheless formed the basis for many of their subsequent interpretations of what it meant, socially speaking, to be handicapped or to have a handicapped person in the family. Parenthetically, we might note that it is probably such feelings of alienation that most distinguish the individual or family crisis from mass disaster, in which, typically, many persons who are known to one another experience like hardships and losses at the same point in time.

In addition to the feeling of having been singled out for misfortune, other alienative elements were imparted to the crisis experience by the social meanings of crippledness in our society and the parents' recognition that the child stood in danger of one day arriving in this category. Having themselves felt pity, or even repugnance, toward crippled persons, they grew uncomfortably aware that the arousal of these sentiments in others in no way aided the crippled person to attain friendships, vocational success, marriage, "a pleasant personality," or the like. The possibility of permanent crippling seemed to them an unjust and unfair hardship—one that threatened to relegate the child to a kind of low-caste status in society. The sense of injustice was conveyed by the metaphors of violence and foul play employed by several fathers in describing the impact of the event—"a body blow," "a kick in the teeth," "hitting a man when he's down," "a punch below the belt."

The child's contracting of the disease, therefore, loomed for the family as a kind of discriminatory barrier in the attainment of important social values; in short, it was "un-American."[23] A strong hint of this is given in the remarks of Mr. Baker:

> A parent oftentimes builds up the future of his offspring. . . . We tell ourselves, "My boy, I can see in him possibilities untold. He's quick minded. He's quick on his feet. He's quick with his hands. There's no telling what he'd grow up and do." My life is formed around watching him grow up. Now, everything that you imagine naturally is through rose-colored glasses. Everything is good. Those are the things that keep people in sanity. If you don't have those things to cling to, . . . you have no purpose here. Why should I be here? It doesn't take long in life for most of us to find out that me, myself, and I are very small. It's what we can dream, what we can build in our own minds, our imagination. Polio kills that. It stops that dream. It cuts it short. . . . If he has a bad leg, he'll never fly. I used to be a flyer in the war. That was very glorifying. It's very self-pleasing, because you're picked out among many. A lot of times you visualize your son following in your footsteps. . . . And when polio enters your mind, that Gerry's not going to be able to fly—maybe he won't be able to be a good 100-yard-dash man, maybe he won't be able to swim as fast as his daddy, play table tennis, ride bicycles. . . . And when you think your boy has polio, all of that flashes through your mind in a split second. As I said, it happens quick what goes through your mind, but it takes a long time to explain it. It takes quite a while.

[23] I am indebted to David Riesman for having originally suggested this analogy to me.

The psychologically alienative character of the crisis experience—in the midst, interestingly, of a rallying of community support for the family—was not without its positive aspect in human terms. Thus, the father who saw in his son's polio the wreckage of his personal "American dream," concluded his statement with: "I'll have to start building my castles over again with Gerry if he has a bad leg. Maybe he won't be able to conform to all these expectations I have built around him." Other parents, perhaps having come to a finer appreciation of human frailty, vowed to be more tolerant and gentle with their children. Many also regarded the experience as a test of their family's solidarity, one that would call forth in family members deeper understanding and greater skill in the management of their relations with one another.

For some, the experience was productive of social and self-insights that less extreme circumstances might not have occasioned. In Mead's words, it helped certain of the families to take "an attitude of living with reference to a larger society."[24] Thus, Mr. Short, through a negative appraisal of his own past behavior, was led to a new appreciation of the bonds joining him to his fellow men. In answer to the question, "How have the neighbors been to the family since this happened?" he replied:

Very, very nice. Extremely nice, in fact. I feel a bit ashamed because last year when the young girl up the street contracted polio, my first thought was, "Eddie hasn't been playing with her, has he?" That was my first question when I walked into the house. My wife said yes, he had been. And yet when this happened to us, everyone around—at least no one has approached me in an abusive manner, in any way sarcastic and nasty. They've all been overly nice, very nice. . . . And, as I said before, it makes me feel a bit ashamed that the fearsome thought came to my mind that Eddie had been playing with her. Of course, they may have had the same reaction initially when this happened to us. But they got over it and then came around and asked if they could help.

Finally, a few parents seemed to derive from the crisis experience and their pained involvement in it—"You can talk about it all you want, but unless it strikes home it's not the same thing," many of them

[24] G. H. Mead, *Mind, Self and Society,* Chicago: University of Chicago Press, 1934, p. 217.

remarked—an awareness of the superficial, largely evasive character of many of the conventional expressions of sympathy and concern extended to those in distress. The discovery that they themselves had resorted to these socially acceptable, though shallow, devices—perhaps from an aversion to involvement in the burdens of others—had a disquieting effect on their appraisal of themselves as human, as distinct from sociable, beings.

Whether the insights evoked by the crisis experience were more than fleeting and ultimately unassimilable fragments of novel experience is difficult to assess. In view of our great ignorance of the meaning and breadth of this kind of inner experience, it would seem unwise to conclude that they were of little or no account.

SUMMARY

Although varying from family to family in temporal and circumstantial details, the crisis experience in the 14 families studied revealed a common perceptual-interpretative pattern. This consisted of a series of definitions and redefinitions by the parents of the meaning of the child's symptoms, each successive definition placing greater cognitive strain on the commonplace diagnoses (e.g., a cold, upset stomach, the flu) first made by them to explain his illness. However reluctantly, and despite much vacillation, in time they abandoned this explanatory framework, with its "routine plausibility," adopting in its place an emergency definition of severely threatening proportions—i.e., that the child had polio.

This process—which, incidentally, appears to be generic to a wide range of crises and disaster situations—can for purposes of analysis be broken down into successive stages of development. Following in large part the terminology used in mass-disaster research, I have called these stages prelude, warning, impact, and inventory.

In the prelude stage, the family exists in a state of relative equilibrium, content to view the illness as an ordinary ailment of childhood. Such unusual symptoms as appear are unattended to or, if recognized, assimilated easily within this diagnostic scheme.

As a rule, the warning stage commences with some dramatic symptomatic or behavioral occurrence: e.g., the child falls for no apparent reason, cannot raise himself from bed, or is unable to move his leg. This poses a severe challenge to the simple diagnosis that the family has previously been entertaining. Even at this stage, however, it is not uncommon for them to explain the occurrence so that it somehow is compatible with their initial, benign diagnosis of the child's illness. At the same time, however, enough doubt and fear are generated for them to initiate a course of action (e.g., calling a doctor, taking the child to a hospital) that eventuates in a medically authoritative diagnosis of paralytic polio.

Despite the reluctance of many of the parents to accept the diagnosis, its mere proclamation is of such great moment as to elicit the extreme reactions of fear, grief, and loss that constitute the impact stage. Following the abatement of this condition is the inventory stage, a period of stocktaking, reappraisal, and initial attempts to formulate perspectives for the long recovery phase. Although certain alienative features emerge in the inventory stage—chiefly the family's sense of having been singled out for misfortune and detached from a universe of "normal" experience—for some the period is also productive of novel re-evaluations of the self and of one's bonds with one's fellow man.

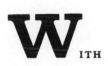
WITH

Chapter 3. Perspectives on Recovery: The Child in the Hospital

the polio victim's admission to the hospital, the crisis enters a new and very different stage. No longer do things simply "happen" to the family in a seemingly random and purposeless way. Hospitalization represents plan, purpose, and order, the introduction of an institutional scheme within which private hopes and fears take on new meaning.

I have called this stage "recovery," although it encompasses much more than the kind and degree of bodily recovery experienced by the sick child in the succeeding months. The child's removal from the home and its effects on him and on the family; the family's developing relationship with the largely unfamiliar world of the hospital; and the community's attitude toward the family are all of interest to us.

In this chapter and the next, therefore, we shall consider how the process of recovery came to be conceived by the sick child and his family, and how their conceptions were modified in the course of their developing relationship with the hospital treatment system and its agents. This chapter will deal with recovery orientations during the period of hospitalization,[1] and Chapter 4 will consider alterations in these orientations following the child's return home.

[1] Duration of hospitalization for the 14 children varied from two to seven months, the mean being five months.

47

So as to understand more fully some of the medical contingencies affecting recovery from polio and their relevance for the interaction of family and hospital, it is necessary first to digress briefly into a discussion of the pathology of spinal poliomyelitis.

PATHOLOGY AND PROGNOSIS IN SPINAL POLIOMYELITIS[2]

The key pathological fact in spinal poliomyelitis is the damage or destruction sustained by the large motor cells of the spinal cord as a result of the pathogenic action of the polio virus. As part of the central nervous system, the spinal cord is, among other things, the innervating seat of the various motor functions of the body. The polio virus may attack any of the great number of cells contained in the spinal cord and brain stem, but it has a special affinity for the large motor cells located in a vertical subsection of the spinal cord known as the anterior horn. These are the cells that innervate the skeletal muscles of the body—those of the arms, legs, abdomen, chest, and neck. Damage to or destruction of the anterior horn cells of the spinal cord gives rise, therefore, to temporary or permanent paralysis of the corresponding skeletal muscles. Deprived of innervation, the affected muscles lose tone, become flaccid, and, depending on the amount of damage sustained by their corresponding cells, eventually undergo such secondary degenerative changes as shrinkage and atrophy. Return to normalcy in the muscles occurs only if, when, and to the extent that the cells recover and re-establish innervation:

> Cells which have been destroyed . . . can never be reproduced. Cells which have been damaged but not destroyed may recover their physiologic function. If all the [cells] which innervate a particular muscle have been destroyed, that muscle will be completely and permanently paralyzed. If some of the cells have been killed and some survive there will be a partial recovery of the power of the muscle, the degree, naturally, being dependent on the relative number of the motor cells which recover. If all the cells remain vital after the destructive phase of the

2 The source of nearly all the material in this section is the American Orthopaedic Association, "Infantile Paralysis, or Acute Poliomyelitis: A Brief Primer of the Disease and Its Treatment," *Journal of the American Medical Association*, CXXXI (August 24, 1946), 1411-19.

disease has run its course, there is the possibility of a return of normal power in the muscle.[3]

It should be noted, further, that medical science has discovered no way of arresting or lessening the severity of the viral attack on the horn cells once it has begun; nor has it found a way of treating the damaged cells so as to restore their muscle-innervating potential, in whole or in part. According to all evidence, such recovery as occurs in the damaged cells is spontaneous.

The central prognostic problem in spinal poliomyelitis then, is: how badly damaged are the large anterior horn cells of the spinal cord, and what are the chances that they will spontaneously regain their muscle-innervating potential? Since there is no direct way of assessing these matters with a living polio patient—dissection and laboratory examination of spinal tissue would be required—the condition of the affected muscles themselves (their strength, tone, flaccidity, etc.) at specified times following the acute attack serves as an index of the damage sustained by the motor cells of the anterior horn and as the basis for estimating the likelihood of their recovering their function. Prognosis in these matters is based not on known laws of cellular deterioration and regeneration but on years of accumulated clinical experience in matching inferences of probable muscle recovery with systematic observations of the muscular state of the patient following the acute phase of the disease. Inadequate as such knowledge may seem from a theoretical standpoint, its predictive value should not be underestimated. Much more often than not, the estimates made by the doctor and the physiotherapist of the degree to which the patient's muscle capacity is likely to return prove accurate. While few, if any, practitioners would be so rash as to rule out completely the possibility of important uncertainty factors in this connection, this is not the same as total ignorance of the probabilities.

Estimates of this kind are made, as a rule, some six weeks to three months following the onset of the disease, on the basis of a series of careful and extensive muscle examinations made periodically on the patient from the time of his admission to the hospital. The contingen-

3 *Ibid.*, p. 1414.

cies governing prognosis at this point are, in general, of the following order:

> Muscles that [have shown] early and rapidly developing return of strength will probably make a full recovery. Those which have but moderate or little strength at the end of this period will probably never make complete recovery. Muscles which are completely paralyzed at the end [of this period] will probably always remain so. In other words, at the end [of this period] the spinal motor cells have or have not recovered their physiologic activity and no further change in them may be expected.[4]

On the basis of such estimates, treatment—particularly the physiotherapeutic regime—is planned and administered during the ensuing months of hospitalization and in many cases for a considerable period following hospitalization. In general, the convalescent treatment of poliomyelitis is planned to accomplish one or more of the following objectives—depending, of course, on the condition of the patient at the end of the six-week-to-three-month period.

1. *With muscles evidencing complete or near-complete return of potential*: therapeutic prophylaxis of such potential through a balanced regime of bed rest, exercise, and most important, through the maintenance of good over-all bodily health. With these muscles, little active treatment is called for.

2. *With muscles evidencing partial return of potential*:

   a. strengthening of the less damaged portions of the muscle or muscle group so that they may safely assume a greater than normal burden in the functioning of the whole muscle group. For example, in the case of a muscle that is 70 per cent destroyed and 30 per cent viable, it is frequently possible through a long regime of physiotherapy to strengthen the viable portion so that it can assume 50 or 60 per cent of the muscle's normal functioning. Rarely, however, can muscles more than slightly denervated be brought to anything approximating full normal functioning.

   b. In addition, or alternately, depending on the site of the paralysis, undamaged muscles or muscle groups adjacent to

[4] *Ibid.*

damaged ones can sometimes be trained and strengthened to compensate for the lost muscle functioning.

3. *With important muscles or muscle groups whose denervation is such as to result in complete, or virtually complete, loss of function in the affected part (e.g., inability to raise the leg, rotate the ankle, bend the knee)*: physical training and preparation of the patient for the use of supportive appliances (braces, crutches, orthopedic shoes, pelvic bands) to aid him in compensating for the loss of normal motor and ambulatory functioning.

Other medical considerations, too specific to discuss here, influence the treatment plan set forth by doctors, particularly for patients who have sustained a more than minor loss of muscle capacity.

With an eye to topics to be considered later in this chapter and in the next chapter, we might summarize the foregoing as follows:

1. The polio virus attacks the muscle-innervating cells of the anterior horn of the spinal cord, not the secondarily affected muscles themselves or the nerve fibers leading to them.

2. Although uncertainty factors to some extent becloud prognoses on the post-convalescent functional capacity of the patient, treatment personnel can frequently make reasonably good over-all prognoses some six weeks to three months following onset of the disease.

3. Finally, in no sense is the patient "cured" of spinal poliomyelitis; that is, there is no known direct treatment that can restore the damaged or destroyed muscle-innervating cells. Whatever restoration occurs in these cells is spontaneous *(vis medicatrix naturae);* nothing can be done to hasten or complete the process. In those many cases, therefore, in which cellular regeneration is only partial or does not occur, recovery, medically speaking, consists wholly in the patient's developing, with or without external supports, substitute or compensatory skills for overcoming as much of his functional loss as possible.

CHANGING RECOVERY ORIENTATIONS[5]

In a very real sense, poliomyelitis casts the sick child and his family into a new world, quite different from that to which they are accustomed. The child's paralysis not only affects his ability to manipulate

[5] See Fred Davis, "Definitions of Time and Recovery in Paralytic Polio Convalescence," *American Journal of Sociology,* LXI (May, 1956), 582-87.

his body but also severely alters his customary motor relations with significant persons and social objects. In a great many cases, the victim cannot walk for several months following the acute attack. He is taken away from family and playmates and set down in strange surroundings where the routine is unfamiliar and where those who minister to him change with great frequency. No longer is he the only child or one among several; he is one among many. Generally, he has only the vaguest idea of what is being done to him or why. When he entered the hospital, 11-year-old Marvin Harris said later, "I didn't know what they were going to do. I didn't know what they were going to feed us, or what they were going to let us do—stand up or sit, or let us see our mothers, or something like that. I didn't know what they were going to do."

For the parents, too, many unknowns suddenly loom. Apart from their primary concern over the child's condition and anxiety regarding the outcome of his illness, they are bewildered by the numerous hospital rules and regulations that intervene to deny them their customary access to and control over him. The exercise of normal parental responsibility for the child is largely removed from their hands and placed in those of strangers.[6] Whereas formerly they could summon or approach the child at will, they now are "permitted to visit" once or twice a week. In the receiving hospital, where the sick child spends 10 to 14 days before transfer to a convalescent hospital, they are not even allowed to come close to him. Because of hospital rules regarding contagion, they must speak to him from behind a glass partition. At this stage, many of the parents can barely conceive of being without the child, much less of the child's being without them. Said Mrs. Manning: "I feel like I should be down there with her, helping her, and if she wants anything I could be there to give it to her; and I can't be there. And it gives you a not very good feeling."

In short, both the child and his parents require definition of the procedures and purposes of this unfamiliar world into which they have been thrust and of its relationship to the everyday world with which they are familiar. Most urgently in need of definition in their eyes are,

[6] Cf. Joseph Greenblum, "The Control of Sick-Care Functions in the Hospitalization of a Child," *Journal of Health and Human Behavior*, II, 1 (Spring, 1961), 34.

of course, the controlling questions of recovery and length of stay in the hospital. At this early stage of hospitalization, treatment personnel are bombarded incessantly with the same questions: How will he come out of it? How long will he have to stay?

Except in the infrequent case of an unusually rapid spontaneous recovery, doctors and physiotherapists offer no answers to these questions at this time. As was pointed out earlier, the assessment of relatively permanent muscle damage, upon which prognoses regarding the extent of muscle recovery are based, cannot be made until six weeks to three months following the acute attack. For this reason the doctors at the receiving hospital scrupulously avoid making predictions of any kind and merely try to "handle" the family's inquiries as best they can.

Despite the doctors' refusal to answer questions at this time, a number of situational factors combined typically to lead the family to fashion a rudimentary perspective on recovery. As we shall see, this was at variance in major respects with the recovery perspective implicit in the course of the disease and the hospital's treatment regime. Chief among the factors influencing the family's perspective was the human proclivity to supply answers to urgent questions. Thus, when the receiving hospital doctors offered little but neutral answers to questions of recovery and outcome, parents frequently drew their own conclusions. Interestingly, even the doctors' refusal to offer prognoses was given a positive interpretation by many parents. Expecting doctors to be cautious and conservative in their estimates, the parents often turned to their own psychological advantage this familiar reluctance of doctors to "stick their necks out." Said Mr. Ellsworth:

> I think that's one reason that maybe I'm more optimistic than my wife or anybody else is now. Because I'll see things that the doctor sees and they'll make me optimistic. But he don't dare be optimistic about them. A doctor would have himself in the middle if he said a patient was going to be all right and it turned around and died or something the next day.

We mentioned earlier that in the inventory stage of the crisis—the same period now being discussed from another vantage point—many parents experienced great relief when they learned that their child was not an iron-lung case or in danger of dying. This, too, helped bring about a relatively optimistic re-evaluation of his condition. Many parents also derived encouragement from incorrect or misinterpreted statistics on paralytic-polio recovery or, more often, from the reassuring reports of friends and neighbors about some ex-polio patient who "came out of it without a mark." The following statements are representative of the many optimistic appraisals elicited from parents during the first weeks of the child's hospitalization:

Mrs. Short: I feel that it will take time, but I feel that he will recover. I strongly feel that he will. [*Interviewer:* How long, would you say?] Oh, I'll say it'll take from two to three months to get him back on his feet completely. I feel that. I don't really know too much about polio.

Mrs. Mason: Well, I'm hoping and praying that she'll come out without any mark at all. I've heard of two cases and I'm putting my hopes on that too. A little boy here that the preacher was telling me about, a couple of years ago he had polio. He goes to Sunday school, and they say—I haven't seen the child—I intend to go up and talk with the mother and I want to see the little boy. But they said he had a bad leg and they say now you can't notice it, except if he runs. . . . Also, someone was telling me that someone they had known had come out of it all right. You would never know that he had polio if someone wouldn't tell you that he did.

Mrs. Harris: I think that Marvin is going to walk just as good as he did before. . . . If he had to go into the iron lung, I don't think I'd be feeling that way. But things the doctor has told me, that he doesn't think it'll go any further . . . so I feel like it's just that leg, and it's a wonderful thing the work that they do with children now. I feel like Marvin'll walk and he'll walk just as good as he ever did.

The ideational components of this early recovery orientation may, in general, be categorized as follows: (1) a short-term time perspective regarding the duration of hospitalization and recovery, the former usually extending to no more than two or three months and the latter rarely to more than six months; (2) a rather undifferentiated concept of the nature of progress in recovery in which few, if any, intermediate steps are anticipated (e.g., it was thought that the child would be "up and walking soon"); (3) an expectation that the child will either recover fully or, if not, that he will escape being handicapped to any significant extent.

Except for one family,[7] this early recovery orientation underwent important changes during the first month or so of the child's hospitalization. First, the time perspective on hospitalization and recovery became lengthened. Next, the concept of progress in recovery became more differentiated and gradualistic. Finally—although this was most resistant to change—the anticipation of a more or less perfect outcome gave way to qualification and in general assumed a much more contingent and problematic aspect. These changes can be seen by comparing the above quotations with those that follow, made by the same parents a month or two following the child's admission to a convalescent hospital.

Mrs. Short, who thought her son would be back on his feet in two to three months:

> Well, I had to get used to it all over again from what I expected from the beginning. Because I never expected for him to have had it as bad as he did. I just thought he was a mild case. And I kind of felt, well, that he would be up and around in at least three months. But I don't expect that now. I think he'll probably be there six months or a year, something like that. Like they say, because it's a slow recovery and that's the way it's done.

Mrs. Mason, who drew great encouragement from stories of the complete recovery of two ex-polio victims:

> She was hurt a whole lot more than I thought she was. I mean, I felt— good Lord, I thought by this time she'd be completely well and that we would hardly know that she had it. But it'll take a long time, and then we're not too sure about her left leg.

Mrs. Harris, who took her son's not having to go into an iron lung as a sign that "he'll walk just as good as he ever did":

> I don't say that I expected him to be walking around, but I never thought that they'd keep him laying down all the time. It's over two

[7] The Bakers, whose son made an unusually rapid spontaneous recovery and spent a total of less than two months in both the receiving and convalescent hospitals.

months! . . . I thought he'd at least be sitting in a wheelchair, you know. But I guess if I want him to be well and walking again, I guess that's what he has to go through. . . . It just seems endless, like I'll never see him sitting up.

How can we account for these changes? From a simple, common-sensical point of view it might be argued that they are but the direct reflection of the changes in physical condition and morale exhibited by the child during his hospital convalescence—i.e., a self-evident estimate derived from self-evident data.[8] This position is naïve, however, in that it fails to take account of the important definitional influences deriving from the family's interaction with doctors and other treatment personnel once the child becomes subject to the hospital's treatment system. Moreover, as we shall see, rarely in this treatment system is the child's condition at any given time so self-evident as to permit the parents to make clear-cut, unproblematic inferences about his improvement, much less his future prospects. The disappointment of their initial expectation that they would be able to appraise the child's condition, at least roughly, merely by looking at him or by asking him how he felt underlies to a large extent the changes we have noted in the family's recovery perspective.

A more sophisticated explanation of the changes in recovery orientation might hold that initially the parents have great need to resort to optimistic ego defenses that fall away as the family gradually adjusts to the reality of the child's condition. Although it cannot be

---

[8] This view is related to the popular notion that recovery is a more or less spontaneous process that seldom requires definition or explanation, since the patient whose condition is improving "feels better" and "shows it." No doubt it was with some such implicit "philosophy" that the parents in our study first attempted—to their subsequent disillusionment—to assess the progress of and prospects for the child's recovery. With many illnesses and ailments this would seem to be a valid, if oversimplified, approach. With numerous others, however (e.g., mental illness, diabetes, various cardiac conditions, and paralytic polio), this approach affords little enlightenment or reassurance. What distinguishes this latter class of pathological conditions is that the patient's state upon the completion of treatment is, as a rule, very different from what it was prior to the onset of his illness. Therefore, "recovery" from these illnesses tends to undergo redefinition and to become assessed according to criteria very different from those used in the case of a bad cold, for example, or even pneumonia. Without the explanations provided by treatment personnel and the labeled, though frequently esoteric, "proof of progress" built into the treatment regime as such, the patient suffering from polio or a similar disease would have little means of sensing progress or of learning that he is getting better.

denied that many of the family's early estimates function in part as morale-boosting devices, this explanation still begs the question. Whose definition of reality, one might ask—the family's, the hospital's, or some blend of the two? The postulation of a self-generating and self-fulfilling mode of reality adjustment fails to comprehend the interactional process in which "reality" is fashioned. "Reality," in this view, is conceived as an *a priori* essence rather than as a social emergent.

It is our contention that the hospital and its treatment procedures are the agents that reshape and redefine the recovery orientations of the family. This is not to say that hospital definitions are taken over by the family *in toto* through a simple process of displacement of its own definitions. The different settings and demands of the two social worlds inevitably give rise to strain and conflict. This results, as we shall show, in recovery perspectives that are neither precisely those of the treatment regime nor those with which the family began. In an attempt to explicate this proposition and to show how the parent-child-hospital relationship brings about alteration in recovery perspectives, I shall examine separately the component parts of this three-fold tie: the parent and the hospital, the child and the hospital, and the parent and the child. Where appropriate, I shall indicate how events in one relational sphere may augment or counteract those in another.

THE PARENT AND THE HOSPITAL

For the parents, by far the most important factor influencing their changed perspective on the duration, progress, and outcome of the child's treatment is their interaction with hospital personnel as they seek to gain information on these points. In general, the behavior of the parents in these encounters may be characterized as eager, deferential, and subordinate; that of hospital personnel, especially the doctors, as brusque, noncommittal, and superordinate, even at times —or so it appeared to parents—condescending or indifferent. Mrs. Short's account of her conversations with the physicians at the convalescent hospital reflects a typical experience:

> Well, they don't tell you anything hardly. They don't seem to want to. I mean, you start asking questions and they say, "Well, I only have

about three minutes to talk to you." And then the things that you ask, they don't seem to want to answer you. So I don't ask them anything any more.

Among the reasons for this characteristic quality of the interaction between parent and hospital physician is, first, the inherent power discrepancy in the doctor-patient relationship. Little need be said of this oft-noted point except to repeat Parsons' observation that when a patient places himself in the hands of a doctor, he and his family in effect relinquish all *technical* jurisdiction for his treatment and somatic recovery.[9] Secondly, but certainly of no less importance, the bewildering aspect of the hospital bureaucracy, with its grossly disproportionate ratio of patients to doctors, its constant changes of personnel, and its seemingly complex hierarchy of authority, tends to aggravate the parents' sense of having failed to elicit from the staff what they consider relevant and useful information.[10]

Perhaps the most important factor, however, is one that has been noted: There is little that the doctors can tell the parents during the first six weeks to three months of hospital convalescence. To the parents' repeated inquiries—"How long will it be? How will he come out of it?"—the doctors can reply only with such remarks as: "We'll have to wait and see," "Only time will tell," and that standard evasion, "He's doing as well as can be expected."

Although in the beginning the doctor's definition of recovery as a course of uncertain outcome did not appear to alter greatly the parents' hopes—and, for many, expectations—for a more or less perfect recovery, it nonetheless laid the groundwork for a significant lengthening of their time perspective and a refocusing of their ideas on the nature of progress toward recovery. I speak of laying the groundwork because, however likely the parents were to accept the doctor's words as authoritative, their failure to extract from him what they judged to be definitive and meaningful reports usually led them on an information-seeking expedition, both within and without the hospital. This

[9] Talcott Parsons, *The Social System,* Glencoe, Ill.: Free Press, 1951, pp. 441-42.

[10] Cf. Eliot Freidson, *Patients' Views of Medical Practice,* New York: Russell Sage Foundation, 1961, pp. 41-56.

constant bane to the practitioner's control of his client is commonly termed "shopping around."[11]

"Shopping around" within the hospital usually consisted of the parents' taking their questions to physiotherapists, nurses, and sometimes other parents whom they met on visiting days and who, they felt, might be more knowledgeable than they themselves were. When they learned that other parents were equally in the dark, they began to realize that they were not the only ones with whom the doctors were close-mouthed. As one mother (Mrs. Lawson) explained:

> They [the doctors] just hedge more or less, and I've noticed they've done that with other parents too. One other man out there said that he just got discouraged when he talked to a doctor. . . . And one mother out there said to me, "Gee, they told me they couldn't tell me a thing until he'd been here about three or four months." And I said, "Well, my son's been here practically three months and I haven't heard a thing yet."

As for the nurses, it is one of the foremost obligations of their position not to divulge diagnoses and prognoses to the patient or his family, this being a prerogative reserved exclusively for the physician. Beyond such conventional pleasantries as "he's doing fine" and "he's coming along nicely," they limit their exchanges with the family to matters concerning the patient's daily life on the ward. Some of the parents were aware of this and did not attempt to extract information from the nurses. The others soon came to realize that the nurses would furnish them with, as they were given to exclaim in frustration, "nothing I can't learn from the child himself." Mrs. Stewart, who had this experience, remarked: "I don't ask her condition with the nurses any more. . . . They just come around and jolly with you. Maybe they'll give you the time of day, or something like that."

Whatever information about the child's condition the parents were able to gather during the first months usually came from their contact with the physiotherapist, but gains here too were limited. Unlike the rotating interne or resident, who often had no clear memory of the child and had to consult his chart before making a cautious pronounce-

11 See E. C. Hughes, *Men and Their Work*, Glencoe, Ill.: Free Press, 1958, pp. 140-41.

ment to the parents, the physiotherapist as a rule had intimate knowledge of the child's condition through daily contact with him. But, like the doctor, he tried to avoid making prognoses or going into detail with the parents before the end of the six-weeks-to-three-months period. His circumspection with parents was doubtless also related to his unenviable position as someone "in the middle." What he could tell the parents might conflict with what the doctor had told them or excite expectations that he would prefer to leave unaroused. Even though some doctors tended to "pass the buck" to the physiotherapist, his long-acquired sensitivity to the structure of authority in the hospital caused him to resist or deflect the many questions pressed by parents. As one physiotherapist described the situation:

> Most of them [parents] get the word that we'd rather not have them coming around. A few get through now and then and we have to handle their questions as best we can without telling them too much, partly because we don't know ourselves. It's better if they find out for themselves in a natural sort of way.

That at least some parents do "get the word" is shown by a remark of Mrs. Harris: "I'm afraid to go to the PT too much because I know that they're not supposed to discuss the cases. You're supposed to go to the house doctor."

For parents who, by sheer persistence, did manage to "get through" during these first weeks, the contact with the physiotherapist was not always so unrewarding as the foregoing remarks may suggest. Perhaps partly because of the psychological sensitivity that their close work with patients entails, perhaps in part because of the still somewhat marginal status of their profession,[12] the physiotherapists encountered in the study seemed to have superior techniques for "handling the family."

---

[12] Like other ancillary medical specialties, physiotherapy has had to struggle to win a legitimate place in the treatment of certain illnesses. Among other problems, it has had to differentiate its province from those of the frequently condemned chiropractor and the sometimes disreputable masseur. Although physiotherapy is widely accepted nowadays as a legitimate adjunct to the medical treatment of certain illnesses, in many treatment centers a delicate and sometimes uneasy *modus vivendi* characterizes the relations between doctor and physiotherapist. Precise definitions of respective spheres of therapeutic competence and authority are still in the process of being worked out with the medical profession.

Although these techniques were calculated to sidestep the questions uppermost in the parent's mind—concerning the duration and outcome of the child's recovery—they appeared to give the parents a certain amount of satisfaction and even relief. One such technique was to show the parents the child's muscle chart, explaining which muscles had been affected and, depending on the case, perhaps even indicating in a very general way the motor functions associated with particular affected muscles. At this point nothing was said, of course, about the extent of involvement or chances for recovery. Parents who posed these questions were given much the same answer that they had already been given by the doctor—namely, that it was too soon to tell. But compared to the information they received from the doctors and nurses, what the physiotherapist gave them represented a significant increment for many parents, if only because some knowledgeable person had taken the time to answer their questions in other than a perfunctory way.[13] For many of the parents, contacts with the physiotherapist signified the first cracks in the wall of bureaucratic indifference and evasiveness that they had come to associate with the hospital. As we shall show, this interaction had important implications for the way in which physiotherapy and its practitioners were later viewed by the parents, particularly by those whose children were seriously handicapped.

"Shopping around" for information outside the hospital usually meant consultation with other doctors and talks with new-found neighbors and acquaintances whose children, or whose friends' children, had had polio. Consultations with other doctors were infrequent and seldom satisfactory, since the private practitioner was even less able to prognosticate or offer reassurance than was the hospital doctor. One mother, for example, visited a pediatrician to question him about her son's condition but reported in discouraged tones that he had refused to discuss the case.

Accounts by neighbors and friends of ex-polio patients who had

[13] This is yet another illustration of the familiar sociological observation that an organization (here, the hospital), if it is to maintain effective ties with the community-at-large, must in its functioning be sufficiently imperfect—i.e., flexible—as to allow some of those who use its services to evade or get around those very rules and policies that, in the main, govern the organization's relations with its clientele.

experienced perfect or near-perfect recoveries, although reassuring when the child first entered the hospital, came after a time to seem less meaningful to the parents. They could see little connection between such tales and their child's continuing immobilized condition. Told by treatment personnel that "each case is different," the parents came to realize that the experiences of an ex-patient were not a reliable basis for inferences about their own child.

This inconclusive "shopping around" within and without the hospital served to reinforce the doctor's initial admonition that "much is unknown, and only time will tell." "Time" in this context connoted, of course, a long time.

Certain aspects of the hospital regime also contributed to shifts in the parents' recovery perspective. The fact that they were permitted to visit the child only once or twice a week—a sore point with many of them—in itself imparted an attenuated periodicity to their time perspective. Moreover, as these visits continued, the parents came to realize that they could observe only slight changes, if any, from week to week. This was in line with the doctor's warning that progress must be measured in small increments and that striking changes could not be expected over the short run.

The scheduling of periodic muscle checks, four to six weeks apart, also led the parents, as well as the child, to focus on time points and recovery states in the future, rather than on what was defined for them as the inconclusive present. Said Mrs. Lawson: "I asked the doctor if I should check with him every week—would there be any sense in it, you know? I didn't want to waste his time. And he said, well, he didn't think I should check every week, but I could in about four to six weeks, after he had a muscle check."

The periodicity of visits and muscle checks formed part of what might be called the gradient structuring of the recovery regime, an important factor in altering recovery perspectives that will be considered more fully in a later section.

Problems in the Communication of Prognoses[14]

By this point the parents' understanding of the child's condition and prospects had become roughly congruent with the medical definition. Their time perspective on recovery had been lengthened; they no longer anticipated great progress from one week to the next; and, to some extent at least, they were able to contemplate a less than total recovery from the paralysis.

At the end of this six-week-to-three-month period, we have noted, all the important findings were in, and meaningful and fairly accurate estimates could be made of the type and degree of the child's residual incapacity. By then, uncertainty had been greatly reduced for treatment personnel. Was it also reduced to any significant extent for the parents? Were, for example, the parents of those children whose affected muscles had "shown early and rapidly developing return of strength" told that the child "would probably make a full recovery"?[15] Were the parents of those children whose affected muscles showed "moderate or little return of strength at the end of this period" told that the child "would probably never make a complete recovery"? Perhaps most indicative of the extent to which the prognoses of treatment personnel were conveyed to the family, were the parents of those children whose affected muscles were "completely paralyzed at the end of this period" told that these muscles "would probably always remain so"?

The answer to this series of questions is yes for only those parents whose children were diagnosed to be minimally and—perhaps, more significantly—imperceptibly affected. For all other parents, the uncertainty and doubt of the early convalescent period continued throughout the period of hospitalization. For some, it persisted well into the post-

[14] For a more detailed discussion of topics treated in this section, see Fred Davis, "Uncertainty in Medical Prognosis, Clinical and Functional," *American Journal of Sociology,* LXVI (July, 1960), 41-47. Findings and interpretations closely paralleling those presented here are given by Greenblum, *op. cit.,* 32-38; Bernard Kutner, "Surgeons and Their Patients: A Study in Social Perception," in E. Gartley Jaco, ed., *Patients, Physicians and Illness,* Glencoe, Ill.: Free Press, 1958, p. 391; and Richard H Blum, *The Management of the Doctor-Patient Relationship,* New York: McGraw-Hill, 1960, pp. 125-32.

[15] The quoted passages in this paragraph are taken from the statement of the American Orthopaedic Association given on p. 50.

hospitalization period. Few of these parents were told by treatment personnel that the child would be handicapped to some extent. Nor were they told the contrary. Their questions on outcome were, for the most part, hedged, evaded, rechanneled, or left unanswered, much as they had been during the diagnostic period. By and large, the parents were left to "find out for themselves, in a natural sort of way." Only gradually—in some instances, as much as a year and a half following the child's discharge from the hospital—did most of them come to learn the true extent of their child's impairment.

This avoidance of communication with parents by treatment personnel results from a complex of factors. To begin with, to divulge to the parents that the child will be left with a residual handicap of some kind is hardly a simple, matter-of-fact communication; and the greater the child's probable handicap, the greater the reluctance of treatment personnel to break the news to parents. As we have said, to be crippled is not merely a physical attribute of the person, much as we may hold with the enlightened concept that this is all it should be; in our culture it is also an important social fact about the person, carrying with it numerous social disadvantages. Regardless of whether the doctor and physiotherapist personally share popular attitudes toward the handicapped—and it would seem that they could not do so and still work with them as diligently as they do—they cannot help but be aware of the pervasiveness of these attitudes and act accordingly.[16]

To "act accordingly" in the context of hospital practice is to leave the question of outcome open, to make no predictions one way or the other about the child's future disability, and to avoid challenging or openly discouraging the parents' hopes and expectations for a perfect or near-perfect recovery; in short, to allow the family to "find out for themselves in a natural sort of way," in the belief that they will eventually accept the fact of the handicap and somehow "make the best of it." That sensitivity to the social unacceptability of a handicap plays a part in the evasiveness of treatment personnel is attested to by their forthrightness with parents whose children, it appeared, would be left with only a slight disability—e.g., a barely perceptible limp, an inability to run quite as fast as before. Thus, for example, the doctor

16 Cf. Lois Pratt *et al.*, "Physicians' Views on the Level of Medical Information Among Patients," in Jaco, ed. *op. cit.*, p. 220.

and physiotherapist at the convalescent hospital, prior to discharging Gerald Baker, told his mother that the boy had regained the use of at least 75 per cent of his affected muscle capacity and would in time regain virtually all of it, a prognosis that turned out to be essentially correct.

Medically anticipated outcomes of this type deviate so slightly from social definitions of normal endowment that there is little need to censor the communication of this kind of prognosis to parents. However, a perceptible limp, a lurching gait, and the prolonged use of braces or crutches do deviate sufficiently to introduce pronounced constraint in informing the family that one of these outcomes will probably be their child's lot. Thus, at a much later point in convalescence, the same doctor and physiotherapist who had spoken so openly to the Bakers about their son Gerald's prospects told Mrs. Prince, whose son they knew to be more seriously affected, that they were unsure about David's outcome and what supports or appliances he would require. She expressed her uncertainty with poignancy:

> Well, I'm waiting for the day when Mr. O. [the physiotherapist] says to me, "I think he's going to be perfect." I mean, right now they think—they are not sure. From what I gather in conversations, they feel he will be all right. But they have never given me a definite answer, I mean. And that's what we're waiting for, when they say he will not need a brace or he will not need a support. I mean that in so-and-so many months he will be a normal child. That's what we're waiting for.

This mother's hopes remained in large part unfulfilled; although David did manage to leave the hospital without a brace, some eighteen months later he still walked with a very marked lurch and was being readied for a bone-fusion operation.

The natural reluctance of treatment personnel to dash the hopes of parents is not, however, the only reason for the scanty communication between them. The tendency to "string the family along" is apparently accentuated by the bureaucratized character of the doctor-patient-family relationship in the hospital setting as compared with the typical relationship in private office practice. In the bureaucratized hospital setting, the resident staff doctor is prone to take a narrowly circumscribed view of his professional responsibilities to the family of the patient. Were he to break the bad news of the child's handicapped outcome to the family, he would, as likely as not, have a "weeping and emotional" parent on his hands, a situation that many staff doctors eschew because it is time consuming, difficult to handle, and disruptive of their tightly scheduled routines. Furthermore, since the costs of treatment for the 14 polio children were borne by the National Foundation for Infantile Paralysis and not by the parents themselves, the ward doctors may have felt themselves to be under less compulsion to weigh carefully the long-term implications of telling as against not telling than they might have had they been treating the same patients under the more usual fee-for-service arrangement.

Finally, it should be noted that only four of the fourteen families in the study were middle class, and two of these were lower-middle. The rest were working class. Medical sociologists have observed that the amount of information a doctor gives a patient and the amount of time he takes to explain a diagnosis are influenced by his perception of the patient's socioeconomic status, or rather by the moral and characterological attributes that he associates with one socioeconomic level as compared with another. That is, the higher the patient's status, the more likely the doctor is to attribute to him a capacity to comprehend medical explanations, a desire to know all the facts, regardless of how dire the implications, and an ability to maintain a calm exterior in the face of unfavorable prognoses.[17] The fact that many of the families in the study were working class may thus have contributed to what, on the basis of a close reading of the interview protocols of the parents, can only be interpreted as a woeful lack of information and miscomprehension of the medical facts underlying the child's condition and prospects for recovery.

What is perhaps most interesting regarding the paucity of communication between parent and treatment personnel relates, as I have implied, to the role of uncertainty in the pre- and post-diagnostic periods of convalescence. As we have seen, medically there is a pronounced shift from prognostic uncertainty to certainty after the first six weeks to three months following the onset of the disease. Yet nothing approximating a commensurate gain in the parents' knowledge of outcome

17 *Ibid.,* p. 226.

probabilities occurred then or for a considerable period thereafter. Thus "uncertainty," a real factor at the beginning of polio convalescence, came more and more to serve social-managerial ends for treatment personnel. Instead of openly confronting the parents with the prognosis—by then a virtual certainty—that the child would be left with a disability, treatment personnel sought to cushion its impact by hedging, evading questions, and acting as if the outcome were still uncertain. Thus they tried to spare themselves the emotional scenes that outright utterance of the prognosis would probably have entailed.[18]

I raise these points because Parsons, in his otherwise excellent discussion of the doctor-patient relationship, states that much of the strain associated with that relationship can be attributed to the frequent presence of clinical uncertainty.[19] Without taking serious issue with this fundamentally plausible point, we must at the same time not lose sight of the possibility that in many illnesses, especially those of a chronic or permanently incapacitating nature, "uncertainty" is to some extent feigned by the doctor for the purpose of gradually—to use Goffman's very descriptive analogy—"cooling the mark out," i.e., getting the patient ultimately to accept and put up with a state-of-being that initially is intolerable to him.[20]

Before we turn to a discussion of the child in the hospital, it may be useful to summarize some of the functions served by the noted alterations in the parents' recovery perspectives, both for themselves and for the hospital's treatment system. As a result of these changes in perspective, the parents tentatively forego expectations of such ultimate states as seeing the child walking again and "leading a normal life" and come to focus instead on such sequentially phased, short-range goals as his sitting up in bed, gaining sufficient strength to move an affected limb, or moving about on crutches. A closer correspondence is thereby engendered between the parents' expectations and the

18 Cf. Davis, "Uncertainty in Medical Prognosis," *op. cit.*, pp. 44-45.

19 Parsons, *op. cit.*, pp. 449-50.

20 Erving Goffman, "On Cooling the Mark Out," *Psychiatry*, XV (November 1952), 456-57. Consider in this connection the "line" sometimes given the patient with a cancer of expected long-term malignancy. Death is, of course, the hardest and most fateful of all statuses into which a patient and his family may have to be "cooled."

pacing of the child's treatment regime. These modifications in the parents' recovery perspective free treatment personnel, particularly the doctor, from repetitive and incessant questioning. Once they come to define recovery as slow and uncertain, many parents begin to feel that there is not much point in "pestering" the busy doctor. Thus relieved to a large extent of the burden of continually having to answer questions and of having to cope with the emotional upset of the family, the doctor can devote himself more fully to what he regards as his primary tasks—diagnosis, prescription, and treatment.[21] Finally—and here I offer without comment the treatment personnel's own view of the matter—postponement and evasion of the socially crucial issue of outcome affords the parents, especially those whose children are seriously handicapped, time to reorganize gradually their attitudes toward the child's altered life situation. The dysfunctional consequences for child and family resulting from this view will be discussed in the next chapter.

THE CHILD AND THE HOSPITAL

A prime prerequisite for structuring and defining the child's recovery orientation in the hospital is the loosening of his affective ties with home and his immersion into the hospital's subculture of illness. If the child feels his separation from parents and home acutely and unremittingly, as he does at the beginning, his incorporation of hospital routines and values is mechanical at best. The passage of each day is keenly felt as but further forced separation from the familiar and loved. In the phraseology of hospital personnel, this child is not "a cooperative patient."

The parents, of course, attempt at first to tell the child why it is necessary for him to remain in the hospital and why he should "listen to the doctors and nurses and be a good patient." These admonitions are usually accepted by the child, sometimes passively and sometimes under protest, but in themselves they can hardly account for his soon

21 Cf. Kutner, *op. cit.*, pp. 395-96.

becoming a "cooperative," even a contented, patient. Rather, it is the hospital itself that accomplishes this by its own devices.

The immersion of the child into the subculture of sickness proceeds on many well-charted fronts.[22] In general, it is facilitated by the restriction of parental visits to one or two a week; by the assumption on the part of personnel of many parental functions; by the duplication on the ward of many of the familiar activities and diversions of the home (e.g., television, games, picture and comic books, group play, etc.); by a reward and punishment system, both formal and informal, which reinforces good behavior and cooperative attitudes as these are defined by treatment personnel; and—most important, perhaps—by the fact of living in a milieu in which illness is the norm rather than the deviation, a condition that permits the child to assimilate the hospital's universe of special meanings, goals, and evaluative rankings.

The transfer of the child from the receiving hospital to the convalescent hospital plays an important part in this socialization process. While in the receiving hospital the child is in pain much of the time and, because of the danger of contagion, is kept in isolation. When his parents visit, he can speak with them only from a distance, separated from them by a glass partition. He may be kept on a liquid diet. All this tends to intensify the homesickness and feelings of isolation that hospitalization in itself arouses.

By comparison, life in the convalescent hospital seems much less deprived. By the time the child arrives there, he is usually out of pain. He is placed in an open ward with children his own age with whom he can talk and play. Games, movies, and television are provided. A schoolteacher, an occupational therapist, and various volunteer workers visit his bedside daily. On visiting days his parents can come directly up to him and do not have to talk at a distance.

The pleasures of sociability after the days of isolation have a telling effect on the children and contribute much to their positive involvement in the treatment regime.[23] Soon after their child entered the

[22] For a parallel account of how this occurs among adult, long-term patients, see Renée Fox, *Experiment Perilous,* Glencoe, Ill.: Free Press, 1959, pp. 139-81.

[23] For a considerably more skeptical view of the psychological effects of hospitalization on children, see James Robertson, *Young Children in Hospitals,* New York: Basic Books, 1958, pp. 19-28.

convalescent hospital, most of the parents commented on how much happier he was and how much his morale had improved. The children voiced similar feelings:

Interviewer: How do you feel now compared to the way you were feeling at Eastern Hospital?

Marvin Harris: Much better.

Interviewer: In what way?

Marvin: Well, we have more things to do, watch television, boys come in and talk to you, and have more fun.

Interviewer: Any other ways that you're feeling better?

Marvin: Well, your mother can kiss you, or give you things, come in and everything. And over at Eastern she couldn't.

It is against this background of loosened, although by no means severed, affective ties with home that the requisite changes in the child's recovery orientation are brought about. As in the case of the parents, the child's time perspective is lengthened, and his concept of progress toward recovery takes shape and becomes more gradualistic in its scope. Whatever concern he feels about his ultimate outcome is to a remarkable degree (much more so than is true of the parents) laid aside, repressed, or suppressed.[24] The following observations made by two of the physiotherapists who treated some of the 14 children testify to these points:

When they come in here, the children think in terms of days. Very soon they're thinking in terms of weeks and not long after that in terms of months.

Like other kids his age [five years old] I don't think he thinks about being crippled or disabled, or knows what it means. That strikes them when they get home and meet normal kids again. Here everyone is sick and he feels more fortunate than others he sees around.

[24] That there existed at least suppressed concern about outcome is attested by many of the responses the children made on the psychological projectives administered to them. For example, a recurrent theme running through their stories on the Children's Apperception Test was that of the sick animal hero who, because he obeyed the doctor and his parents, recovered and was then able to join all the other animals in play.

Two facets of the change in the children's recovery perspective must be considered in particular. The first is what I earlier termed the gradient structuring of the physiotherapy regime, and the second refers to the informal group processes on the ward by which the children came to acquire much significant, though not always accurate, information about their illness and the treatment regime.

In general, the gradient structuring of the physiotherapy regime involves the child in a step-by-step progression toward what doctor and physiotherapist estimate as optimal motor functioning within the limits imposed by his residual muscular incapacity. This goal, which in many cases falls far short of the ideal of *normal* motor functioning, is masked from the child by the intense concentration that the physiotherapist brings to bear on small, day-by-day gains. At the same time, however, these small, carefully paced advances contribute greatly to the aura of "progress" that pervades the physiotherapy regime. Just as promotion from the second to the third grade signifies for the child successful progress toward the ultimate goal of graduation from school, these small increments in strength and mobility signify progress toward the desired goals of walking, running, playing, and other activity.

The physiotherapy regime, which in its very design faithfully captures the essence of the Protestant ideology of achievement in our culture—namely, slow, patient, and regularly applied effort in pursuit of a long-range goal—has built into it, as it were, its own prophecy of success. Moreover, it is an institutional format with which the child is already familiar from school, playground, and home, a way of attending to the future that runs through many of his prior socialization experiences. Suggestive of this ideational correspondence is the game nine-year-old Johnny Lawson chose to play with the research psychologist in about the sixth month of his stay at Hillside Hospital.

> At this point Johnny introduced me to a game which I believe he made up, or at least modified or condensed from several others. He first drew a ladder with the word GOAL at the top, and then we each drew "men" at the bottom and moved them in turn—more or less as in parcheesi—toward the goal. Of course, he won. The name of this game, Johnny told me afterward, was "Climbing the Rungs."

It is worth noting also how the gradient structuring of the physiotherapy regime tapped the deep and implicit faith of the families in the efficacy of "will power" in overcoming adverse conditions. Not only was the regime attuned (and of course individually adjusted, as required) to the child's exercise of will power, but his progress from stage to stage frequently signified for parents and others that he possessed this highly prized character trait in sufficient measure. In addition, the great amount of activity and application called for in the regime, as well as the elaborate gymnastic-type apparatus employed (dumbbells, wall pulleys, horses, parallel bars, inclined walking ramps, etc.), left little room for doubt that "something was being done," and thus further reassured the family.[25]

By way of illustrating these and other aspects of the physiotherapy regime, consider the case of a child with extensive residual paralysis in one leg that prevents him from standing and walking. The physiotherapist may begin treatment by bending and manipulating the paralyzed leg while the patient lies on a stretcher bed. This procedure not only familiarizes the physiotherapist with the exact site and degree of muscular incapacity but also serves to indicate to the child that the leg is potentially of some use, something that a passive regime of bed rest might not make evident so early. Several days later, the child may be suspended for the first time in the hydrotherapy pool, where the buoyant effect of the water permits him to move the paralyzed leg about more easily than he otherwise can. This in itself is a rewarding and pleasurable experience and reinforces the sense of muscle potential. In the course of several months the child may progress from moving the leg to and fro while lying supine upon a mat, to standing up while being held by the physiotherapist, to ambulating up and down a ramp while he supports himself on arm rails, to taking his first tentative steps with the aid of braces and crutches.

As the child masters each stage of the treatment he is prepared by

[25] This is in line with what Parsons (*The Social System, op. cit.,* pp. 466-67) views as the activity bias of American medical practice. It is interesting that while many orthopedists privately doubt that physiotherapy *per se* contributes much beyond what natural recuperative processes themselves can accomplish, few press the point in actual treatment situations because they are aware, implicitly at least, of the valuable psychological functions it serves.

the physiotherapist for the next stage.[26] The progression not only defines his recovery for him but also functions as something of a reward for efforts he has already made. In short, even though his disability might, when viewed by the layman, appear marked, in his physiotherapeutic experiences he learns by word and deed that he is "getting well." This becomes particularly evident when the child learns that he is to be fitted for a brace. The nine children in the study who received braces regarded them not as a sign of severe or permanent incapacity but as proof that they were getting well and were ready to go home. Being fitted for braces was for them but another necessary and welcome *rite de passage* on the road toward full recovery.

Richard Johnson:	I'm going to get my brace soon.
Interviewer:	When did you find out that you might get a brace?
Richard:	Because I'm well.
Interviewer:	Because you're well? Can you tell me about this, Dick?
Richard:	Well, I can bend my legs now, and I got some muscles in them. And pretty soon I'm going to go home, and stay home.

This exchange however, also points up some of the dysfunctional consequences inherent in the easy assimilation by the children of hospital definitions and values. The values of the hospital are not precisely those of the community to which the child will have to return one day. The severely disabled child who, after long treatment, is able to get out of bed and move about on crutches has, in the eyes of the physiotherapist and others in the hospital, made marked and important progress. They encourage the child to share in this conviction. To outsiders—possibly to his parents as well—he may still be just a "poor crippled kid." Thus many parents experienced great shock when they first saw their child walk again, despite the child's obvious pride of accomplishment. Mrs. Manning reported:

> She really walked awful. She just about made it, and it really made me sick because I thought, "Oh, is that the way she's going to walk?" She

[26] For a generic discussion of this type of "coaching" relationship see Anselm Strauss, *Mirrors and Masks, The Search for Identity*, Glencoe, Ill.: Free Press, 1959, pp. 109-18.

could hardly get one leg in front of the other with the brace on. I said, "Oh, Polly, that's fine, you're just doing fine," and she was so pleased. And she said, "Well, I'm going to walk," and she did.

Even more than did their parents, the children learned to peg their expectations around the periodic muscle checks. After exchanging experiences and information among themselves, the children came to believe, for example, that it was at the second muscle check—usually about twelve weeks following admission—that decisions were made about bracing and additional physiotherapy. The muscle checks and other benchmarks on the road to recovery (e.g., being allowed to sit up in bed, being given a wheelchair) became so intimately associated with particular stages of ambulation that the children frequently thought of them as prerequisites for ambulation. As a perceptive eleven-year-old (Geraldine Eaton) remarked somewhat sarcastically, "Nobody around here walks until after they've had their second muscle check."

As much as it helped provide a meaningful framework for the child during his hospital convalescence, the physiotherapy regime still left many important questions of the child unanswered. The child's network of informal relations with other children on the ward furnished the answers to many of these questions, including some on issues so basic that one might assume that no "behind the scenes" clarification was needed. For example, six-year-old Polly Manning, having been told only that her condition required hospitalization, arrived at the convalescent hospital still groping for an explanation of why she was there. It was the girl in the next bed who first provided one.

Polly: The afternoon when I first come in here, then Carol told me and then I knew. . . .
Interviewer: What did Carol tell you about yourself?
Polly: When I first come into here, I said, "Carol, what do I have?" She said, "You have polio."

Carol also told Polly of the physiotherapy treatments that polio children received, who the various children on the ward were, and why they were there. Thus, she gave Polly a category to belong to, told her something about other categories, and pointed out to her who on the ward belonged to which category. The world Polly had just entered assumed at least rudimentary structure for her.

More typically, children explored such questions as "When will I be able to sit up?" "How will I know if I am going to wear a brace?" "When do you get a wheelchair?" "How will I know when I'm due to go home?" They attempted to delineate the telling clues and inter-dependent sequences.[27] The neophyte on the ward was told by the veteran of three or four months what to look for and what kinds of ambulatory advancement and privilege followed certain events and conditions. These predictions came to serve as provisional signposts for the child, who tried to assess their validity by comparing them with what others had told him and what he himself was able to observe. For example, after his second month of convalescence Johnny Lawson announced to the interviewer that he would be going home soon. (Actually, he was not discharged until five months later.) Johnny explained that another boy who had entered the hospital at about the same time and who, according to Johnny, had been "sicker," was then being fitted for a brace. Being fitted for a brace, Johnny had learned from the other children, meant that the boy would be going home soon, and so, therefore, would he.

But, unlike inmates of penal institutions, the children had only the crudest grasp of the contingencies affecting their confinement, so great was the gulf separating their knowledge of their physical condition from that possessed by treatment personnel. As often as not, the estimates of the future developed in the ward milieu proved incorrect.

The deficiency in the body of informal knowledge developed among the children on the ward can be attributed not only to their youth and lack of experience but also to the cultural unavailability to persons in this age group of what might be termed an appropriate institutional model. The children tended to project onto the hospital the image of the only large-scale institution with which most of them were familiar—the school—although a reformatory or disciplinary barracks might prove a more accurate model by which to grasp the confinement contingencies of a hospital population. In the classroom, what hap-

[27] Cf. Julius Roth, *Timetables: Structuring the Passage of Time in Hospital Treatment and Other Careers*, Indianapolis: The Bobbs-Merrill Company, Inc., 1963.

pens to one child by way of instruction, assignments, and promotion more or less happens to all. Hence the oversimplified view of the children on the ward that all "polios" who were there must, because they were labeled "polios," be more or less alike, and that what happened to one would very shortly happen to the others as well.

This took an interesting turn for the children when, after being on the ward for a while, they learned that the class of "polios" was subdivided into "new polios," like themselves, and "old polios," children who, having had polio in the past, were back in the hospital for corrective surgery. The children in the study were perplexed by this situation, and many of them wondered whether they too were fated to return one day as "old polios." Less than a month after seven-year-old Laura Paulus was discharged from the hospital, she told the interviewer that when her polio was "two years old" she would become an "old polio." "Old polios have to go back to the hospital for operations, but I don't ever want to go back to the hospital." (Unfortunately, Laura's residual involvement was so severe that she became an "old polio" even sooner than she feared: 14 months after discharge she returned for a muscle-transplant operation.)

THE PARENT AND THE CHILD

Much has already been said in passing of parent-child relations during the hospitalization period and of their significance for the emergence of recovery perspectives. The loosening of the child's affective ties with home and the affinity of the gradient-like physiotherapy regime with such positively valued concepts as "progress" and "will power" are of primary importance in this connection. A few other miscellaneous considerations also had a bearing on the emergence of recovery perspectives from the context of parent-child interaction.

In an earlier section we showed how the parents' communications with treatment personnel and the rebuffs and disappointments they experienced in "shopping around" materially affected the lengthening of their time perspective. Another significant influence in this direction derived from the appearance of the child during the first weeks of convalescence. Despite their awareness that the child was ill, that he required treatment, and that "it might take a while before he came around," few of the parents were prepared for what frequently met their eyes after the child had been in the convalescent hospital for a week or so.

> *Mrs. Short:* I was a little shocked when I saw the cast on his leg. One week after he was in there they did it. . . . I guess it got my husband worse than it did me. He was really shocked. He said he just stood and looked at first when he saw the cast, and he says he didn't know what went through his mind, but he just thought that—well, he thought maybe they had to operate or something on him.

Such common procedures as putting the child's leg in a cast or placing him in traction and strapping him to a frame in order to inhibit possibly injurious body movement are by no means true indices of the over-all severity of the child's involvement. These procedures are sometimes performed on children with only mild involvement, depending on the kind of muscular imbalance to which the paralysis gives rise. The parents, however, were rarely aware of this or made aware of it by treatment personnel, and the sight of the child's frozen immobility stirred in them visions of more severe involvement than they had imagined.

> *Mrs. Richards:* When you see him strapped down to that frame, it makes you feel kind of sick to your stomach. . . . I don't know exactly what this strapping down is for. . . . I know it's awfully—he's got a strap around his neck and that irritates his neck something awful, and he just can't move! I don't know what it's good for, but I guess it's put there for some purpose. But I would like to know exactly what good it's doing, because if he was able to sit up, I think he'd feel a lot better.

We have noted the relative rapidity with which the once homesick and weeping child became a contented, perhaps even a happy, patient. This, too, had bearing on the development of recovery perspectives by the family. Parents were anxious at first lest the child feel homesick, rejected, and unhappy in the hospital, not only because as parents they were concerned for his happiness, but because they feared that in his misery he would be incapable of harnessing his will power in behalf of recovery. Characteristically, the parents measured the child's adjustment to the hospital by the amount of crying he did when they saw him on visiting days. As this diminished with time, the parents became more convinced that the child was "getting on." Even though he may have wanted to cry, they regarded the mere stifling of tears as a good sign that he was "taking hold" and "putting his mind to getting well."

> *Mr. Prince:* Well, the last couple of times I went there he seemed to be getting used to the idea that he's going to have to stay there until he's able to walk, I mean, get up and sit up. . . . When we leave now he doesn't cry. You can see that he wants to, but he tries his best to fight it off.

The apparent success of the hospital in attending to many of the child's routine needs while simultaneously mobilizing his motivational resources for recovery constituted an important point of leverage in the hospital's exercise of social control over the parents. It served to inhibit possible actions by them that might have undermined the child's morale and close identification with the therapeutic regime. Thus, despite their anxieties about the treatment regime and what the future held for the child, most parents when visiting with the child felt compelled to adopt conventional stances of great certainty and optimism. For example, when her son voiced her own fears that his paralyzed leg was "getting thinner," Mrs. Harris reassured him:

> "Marvin, that's the thing that used to happen before they used to have therapy," I said. "They wouldn't work on children and they just laid there, and from not using it, it would get thinner. But now with that therapy, it's so wonderful for it. They keep it alive, and that doesn't happen to children any more."

As it turned out, Marvin's leg could not be "kept alive"; it did "get thinner."

Finally, as we have noted and will mention again, there was always available to the parents a negative point of reference ("someone worse off") by which they could calculate to advantage their present and, quite possibly, future loss. When the fact of the child's handicap could no longer be evaded or denied, the parents typically turned for consolation to this somewhat abstract scale of human misfortune. "When Mrs. Eaton [another parent in the study] and I happened to pass that ward where they keep the respirator cases, I said to her how lucky we were that our children weren't in iron lungs." So spoke Mrs. Paulus, the mother of the child who turned out to be the most severely disabled in the group, requiring braces on both legs, crutches, a pelvic band, and corrective shoes.

How fragile or serviceable a rationalization this is, it is difficult to say. That it is, however, a significant theme in the problem of self-definition confronting the handicapped child and his family, we shall see in a later connection.

SUMMARY

Beginning with a highly optimistic, short-term outlook on recovery, within weeks of the child's hospitalization the parents came to adopt a much longer time perspective and one that at least permitted them to conceive of outcomes for the child that fell short of full recovery. A complex of cognitive, situational, and structural influences underlay this shift of perspectives. Chief among these were the prognostic uncertainty during the first months of the child's hospitalization, which prevented doctors and physiotherapists from giving parents pertinent information regarding the probable extent of residual handicapping; the loosening of the child's affective ties with home and his immersion in the hospital's subculture of illness; and the gradient-like structuring of the physiotherapeutic regime, which encouraged child and parents to orient themselves to small-step, progressive gains rather than to the distant goal of full recovery.

Although prognostic uncertainty regarding outcome was significantly reduced for treatment personnel by the third month of the child's illness, rarely was the resultant gain in knowledge communicated to the family. This was especially true in cases in which the medically anticipated outcome was relatively poor. Largely because treatment personnel were averse to becoming embroiled in the many delicate socio-emotional issues surrounding crippling, the parents' repeated inquiries on outcome were, even at this late date, met with evasion and hedging. Hospital treatment personnel frequently rationalized this behavior by asserting that the parents would in due time discover for themselves, "in a natural sort of way," that the child was to remain handicapped.

Although this approach may have spared family members some emotional shock, it also perpetuated much misinformation and misunderstanding regarding the course of the disease. As we shall see, this had subsequently adverse effects on the family's ability to implement prescribed rehabilitation measures in the child's behalf.

Chapter 4. Perspectives on Recovery:
The Child at Home

child and family the homecoming was a great event. Regardless of the child's condition or handicap, the recovery outlook of family members took a more optimistic turn when he returned home. A reunion glow suffused the life of the family; doubts were temporarily laid aside, and a determined effort was made to "look on the bright side of things." Several weeks before Laura Paulus was scheduled to be discharged from the hospital, for example, her parents began to make what had formerly been the children's playroom into a separate bedroom for her. The room was repainted and new furnishings and decorations were bought, at considerable expense. The Pauluses and their neighbors then filled the room with gifts and toys with which to welcome Laura—dolls, picture books, a record player, a jewel box, a second parakeet "to keep Laura's old parakeet company," and a multitude of trinkets. Although the family could well have used the extra money, Mrs. Paulus quit her job at a nearby department store in order to get everything ready and then to be able to spend all her time with Laura. Parties, trips, and excursions were planned long in advance. A week before her daughter's homecoming Mrs. Paulus summed up her feelings: "Oh gee, I know one thing! We certainly are much happier now and we're just so glad it's finally coming to an end. . . . I think once she gets back everything'll straighten out all right."

Like honeymoons, however, reunions are of notoriously short duration. The extent to which the parents' optimism was sustained during the months following the child's homecoming depended on a number of factors, chief among them the amount of physical and functional progress the child was able to demonstrate. Such progress as he was to make could no longer be of the spontaneous kind that occurs during the first weeks of convalescence. Rather, it depended primarily on his developing, frequently in a natural and untutored way, compensatory skills by which to overcome to some degree his residual incapacity. As was pointed out in Chapter 3, the development of such skills is in large measure governed by the site and extent of the residual incapacity. From a medical standpoint, therefore, the general proposition can be advanced that the greater the amount and the more functionally strategic the site of the residual incapacity, the less the probability that the child will make significant progress in the post-hospital period.

But, as we have seen, the relationship of the child's residual incapacity to probable progress was rarely brought to the attention of the family before his discharge, especially if the residual incapacity was more than minor. It was at best remotely alluded to or vaguely implied by treatment personnel, but never openly discussed. As a result, many of the parents were greatly misinformed, as the following two quotations illustrate. The first is a report by Norma Jean Mason's doctor to the interviewer several weeks prior to Norma's discharge; the second is a statement made by Mrs. Mason approximately two and one-half months later.

> Maximum improvement has been reached in Norma's case. Any further progress will be minimal. Her leg will remain flail, although operative procedures later on may result in lesser bracing or none.

> It might be three months before they take away that long brace and give her a short one instead. But I'm hoping it'll be sooner than that because Norma Jean seems so much stronger than when she was in the hospital.

Although her remarks at this time were somewhat more cautious than they had previously been, in other portions of the interview Mrs.

Mason continued to speak in terms of her daughter's eventually making a complete recovery. A year later, however, Norma Jean was still wearing her long leg brace, was still using crutches, and, in general, had made little progress since her discharge.

I do not mean to suggest that all or even most of the parents were wholly unrealistic in their expectations. With the lengthened time perspective acquired during the child's hospitalization, they no longer expected too much, too soon. Moreover—and this is an important point to which we shall return later in this chapter—prior to the child's discharge many of the parents *were* told (usually with little explanation) that no further recovery could be expected after a period of twelve to eighteen months from onset of the disease—i.e., roughly six to twelve months following hospital discharge. Thus, they were led at least to contemplate the prospect that the child would not discard his brace or cease limping within mere days or weeks of his homecoming, and that they might have to wait months before this happened. But, as regards the pace and quality of progress he might reasonably be expected to make during this period or its implications for his long-run physical status, the family existed in an informational void almost as great as that present during the first months of convalescence.

What, then, happened to the families' recovery perspectives in the year or so following discharge? Were they further changed, crystallized, or resolved? In order to consider these questions within a meaningful framework, it is necessary to compare the condition of the children at time of discharge with their condition a year or so later.

In Table 1 the patients are classified according to functional capacity: the non-handicapped or minimally handicapped; the moderately handicapped; and the seriously handicapped. These distinctions, as they are used here, not only characterize the child's physical condition at time of discharge and a year later but also relate his condition to his performance and participation in a wide range of activities normal or typical for a child of his age and sex. Hence the term "functional capacity," which takes into account what a person can and cannot do as a result of his handicap and is not narrowly restricted to such purely organic indices as the site and quantitative degree of muscular incapacity or the mere presence of ambulatory anomalies. Not that these are unrelated to questions of performance and participation—obviously they are—but, rather, that in and of themselves they tell us very little about the human costs of a physical handicap.

TABLE 1

Over-all Functional Capacity of the Fourteen Children by Degree of Handicap, at Time of Discharge and Approximately One Year Later

	One Year Later		
At Discharge	Non-handicapped or minimally handicapped	Moderately handicapped	Seriously handicapped
Non-handicapped or minimally handicapped (1)	1	—	—
Moderately handicapped (6)	4	2	—
Seriously handicapped (7)	—	2	5
Total (14)	5	4	5

The category "non-handicapped or minimally handicapped" includes children whose capacity was such that apart from some very minor deficiency—typically, an inability to run as fast as they used to or a slight body sway when negotiating stairs—they could partake in the full round of life common to children of their age group. Such activities as running, playing ball, dancing, hiking, climbing stairs, dressing, washing, toilet care, and attending school were in no way closed to them because of their handicap. Usually the handicap of these children was difficult to detect and became apparent, if at all, only when they were fatigued.

"Moderately handicapped" includes children who could participate in most of but not all the activities listed above. Generally, their impairment extended to such strenuous pursuits as running, playing ball, and hiking, and to the degree that they could participate in these it was frequently necessary for their playmates to adapt the activity to the handicap. Thus, when playing softball, Johnny Lawson was catcher for both sides; when he was at bat, another child ran bases for him. Although all the children in this category wore braces or walked with a decided limp, lurch, or foot drop, they did not give the impression of being severely crippled. In non-athletic activities, they could usually manage to look after themselves with little or no assistance. Body and toilet care presented no serious problems for them, and they could dress, negotiate stairs, and get from place to place with reasonable facility. Some of them could even, after a fashion, run, roller skate, and ride a bike.

Although by no means completely invalided, the children classified as "seriously handicapped" had difficulty not only in physically active pursuits but in sedentary ones as well. Many of them required assistance in washing, bathing, dressing, and going to the toilet. Negotiating stairs or walking any distance usually called for strenuous effort on their part. Even if their playmates altered a game to accommodate them, they were capable of only minor or peripheral participation. When Norma Jean Mason played dodge ball, for example, she would throw the ball from a fixed sitting position while all the other children ran about and took turns being the target; Norma was never the target. All the children in this group wore braces, and many had to use crutches as well if they planned to walk for more than a very short distance. In public they were frequently stared at by strangers. Those who did not attend a school for handicapped children required such special services as pre-arranged transport to and from the school building, help in ascending and descending from street car or bus, classes restricted to the ground floor, and help when going to the school lavatory.

Table 1 shows that a total of six children progressed to a less handicapped category during the year or so in which the families were followed. Four (Sarah Ellsworth, Frank Lee, Geraldine Eaton, and Neil Richards) moved from moderately to minimally handicapped, and two (John Lawson and Edward Short) from seriously to moderately handicapped. These six children and their families will be referred to as the *Progress Group*. Seven of the remaining eight children and their families will be spoken of as the *Stationary Group,* these being children who failed to demonstrate significant improvement in functional capacity during the year or so following discharge. Of the seven, five (Laura Paulus, Marvin Harris, Polly Manning, Norma Jean Mason, and Theresa Stewart) remained seriously handicapped; and two (Richard Johnson and David Prince), moderately handicapped. As we have noted, Gerald Baker and his family belong in a class by themselves in that at the time of discharge Gerald had no residual handicap.

THE PROGRESS GROUP

The improvement in functional capacity characteristic of the six children in the Progress Group began, typically, within weeks after their return home and extended in all cases well into the following year. Particularly in the case of the four children whose residual incapacity at time of discharge was only moderate, the course of recovery was to all intents and purposes completed before the year's end. With all six, the progress demonstrated was apparent and tangible; no careful medical validation or close scrutiny of body movements was required. Activities that they had been unable to perform at time of discharge were for the most part mastered with ease and assurance by the end of the year.

Eleven-year-old Geraldine Eaton, for example, returned home after a three-month hospital convalescence with a perceptible limp and hip lurch. She was restricted greatly in her physical activities, tired easily, and had to nap every afternoon. Her footing was uncertain, and during the first weeks at home she fell several times while moving about the house. Frequently when ascending or descending stairs she assumed a sitting position and bumped along on her buttocks. Otherwise, she was forced to negotiate the stairs very slowly, holding onto the hand rail and bringing both feet to the same step before proceeding to the next. She wore a corrective shoe on her right foot and slept with a splint cast on her right leg. Roller skating and bike riding, two of her favorite pre-polio pastimes, were completely out of the question, and, much to her annoyance and disgust, she was unable to join her playmates in running games.

When seen four months later, Geraldine had made significant progress. Her limp and hip lurch were less perceptible and became obvious only when she was fatigued. She did not tire so easily as she had;

neither did she fall so frequently. She no longer bumped her way up and down stairs, although she still found it necessary to negotiate them slowly, using the halting method described above. Although still unable to roller skate or ride her bike, she could participate to a limited extent in running games. She still used the splint cast when sleeping and wore the corrective shoe on her right foot.

Two months later Geraldine's progress was even more apparent. She could negotiate stairs much more easily and was able to participate fully in running games, although it was by now evident that she would never be able to run as fast as she had before. The splint cast and corrective shoe were no longer required. By this time, Geraldine's limp was perceptible only when she was tired. Tiredness, however, occurred much less frequently. The only remaining incapacity of any significance was her inability to ride a bike.

When she was last seen, a year or so following discharge, this skill too had been mastered. Geraldine's limp was no longer perceptible in the least, although her mother claimed to be able to detect a slight shuffling now and then when Geraldine was tired. She now ascended and descended stairs in a natural fashion, danced, played, and did all the other things typical of a twelve-year-old. According to Mrs. Eaton, all her hopes for her daughter's recovery had been realized. This appraisal had been confirmed at the polio clinic in the previous month.

Characteristically, several things happened to the recovery outlook of the families who were fortunate enough to witness this degree of functional improvement in their children. Most striking, perhaps, was the way in which the rather vague and generalized recovery deadline of twelve to eighteen months posited by treatment personnel assumed for them the quality of a yardstick, divided into equal units of progress. Measured against the intervals of this hypothetical yardstick, the improvement shown by the child, so the parents believed, revealed him to have moved at a faster than normal rate toward the yardstick's terminal point of "complete recovery." As Mrs. Eaton said of Geraldine some six months after her discharge: "Well, I think she's done good! I know they said a year or eighteen months, but I think she's gone faster than that." This is of interest because doctors do not view this time limit in nearly the same way. From clinical experience, they know that some progress of the substitutive or compensatory type does occur after the first six-week to three-month period of spontaneous recovery, its pace and quality depending largely on the site and amount of residual incapacity. This remaining period of approximately 15 months is viewed, then, as a "reasonable time span" within which such compensatory skills may, if the child's condition permits, be developed. After this, additional major improvement can come, in the doctors' view, only from corrective surgery, if such is indicated. Moreover, they claim, the time span of 12 to 18 months from onset is also a "reasonable period" for the family to "adjust to" or "accept" whatever permanent incapacity is to remain with the child. (Fortunately, for the four families whose children moved from moderately to minimally handicapped, relatively little "acceptance" was required.) In no sense, however, do the doctors share the families' conception of this time span as a yardstick on which are demarcated standardized or regularly scheduled increments of functional improvement. Among other reasons, polio cases are much too varied to permit such a measure.

The yardstick conception of time imbued the Progress families' perspective with a sense of accomplishment much like that of the golfer when he "shoots under par" or of the jockey when he makes better than average time for the course. Recovery in this context acquired an "unlimited" connotation. The fact that the child had progressed was taken to mean that he would progress indefinitely, until some magical moment in the future when he would no longer be handicapped, incapacitated, or in any way different from his fellows.

This outlook occasionally engulfed unfavorable facts and probabilities affecting the child's condition of which the family had been at least partially aware earlier. Thus, the Ellsworths—certainly the best-informed family in the study—could plainly see that their daughter's affected leg had grown thinner than her unaffected one, which indicated that a certain amount of irreversible atrophy had taken place. Also, at the time of Sarah's discharge and subsequently, they were told by the hospital doctors that the girl might require surgery in the future to correct certain posture deformities that might result from the partially atrophied extremity. During the months following hospitalization, however, Sarah made good functional progress. She was able to discard her brace, and her limp became less noticeable. In their pleasure and satisfaction over Sarah's progress, Mr. and Mrs. Ellsworth seemed to put completely out of mind—exercising perhaps a more than usual degree of denial—the matter of her atrophied leg and the probability of corrective surgery. The last few times the family was seen the atrophy was never mentioned, and when they were asked about corrective surgery they said that they rarely thought or spoke of it since they did not regard it as very likely. Instead, both parents repeatedly pointed to the progress Sarah had made and reiterated their belief that it would continue well into the future with increasingly good results.

Although with somewhat less certainty, much the same outlook of "recovery unlimited" was demonstrated by the two Progress families whose children had left the hospital in a seriously handicapped condition. When, almost a year after Johnny's discharge, Mrs. Lawson was asked about the possibility of corrective surgery in the future, she stated in somewhat surprised and annoyed tones that "the full improvement period isn't over yet." "Johnny is still improving," she continued, "and as long as he does there won't be anything like that." (Frequently, this is an incorrect assumption in that the improvement the child shows may have no bearing on that part of his condition requiring surgical remedy.) Similarly, until Edward Short was operated on for a tendon transplant a year after his return home—at which time his parents' outlook took a decided downward turn—Mr. and Mrs. Short spoke of how much the child had improved and would continue to improve. Mr. Short even conjectured that the boy might one day play with the local Little League team. As for corrective surgery, Mrs. Short did not expect it to take place until early adolescence (Edward was then eight), if at all.

For the four families in the Progress Group whose children reached a state of minimal handicap, the excelling-the-yardstick perspective on recovery was never demonstrated to be wrong. Although the hypothesis was faulty, it was serviceable in that it allowed parents once again to attribute extraordinary feats of will power and determination to the once badly handicapped child. Said Mrs. Lee, for example, "It was his own wanting to and fighting against it that did it. He'd just talk about when he come home he was going to ride his bike, and, by gosh, he did."

In small ways these incidents add to our culture's ample storehouse of myths, tales, and "known instances"[1] of man's triumphing over seemingly impossible circumstances to prove that it is he and he alone who fashions his fate. The improvement shown by these children became for the parents a miniature re-enactment of the classic American success story.[2] Mrs. Richards, for example, compared her son to "a fellow down in Virginia my husband was telling me about. He had polio and the doctors told him he'd never be able to get out of his wheelchair again. But he did, and he can walk with just a little bit of a limp. And he got married, too. And he didn't have anybody to help him. He just made up his mind he was going to do it himself."

THE STATIONARY GROUP

The seven families whose children remained functionally stationary during the year following discharge present a very different picture. It is not that these children showed no improvement—all of them in time acquired greater strength and proficiency in coping with their handicap—but the improvement they showed did not effect a fundamental advance in their over-all functional capacity.

The case of ten-year-old Norma Jean Mason, a seriously handicapped child, is fairly typical in its general outlines. After a six-month

[1] Franklin D. Roosevelt's life is the most prominent example.

[2] Particularly as regards the goal-directed efforts of children, it may be that our culture systematically exaggerates the difficulty of circumstances, so that the individual soon acquires—rather inexpensively—a "sense of accomplishment in the face of adversity." Perhaps this kind of emotional pump-priming is necessary in contemporary America if the plentiful rewards of our society are to continue to be regarded as rewards. It may be the culture's way of maintaining a sense of ideological continuity with earlier eras of Protestant asceticism and scarcity, when the fewer material rewards available were much harder to come by. What at first, therefore, seems like a significant vestige of "inner-direction" in the generalized American character may on closer examination reveal itself to be little more than a charade. This may in part account for the widespread popularity of such radio and television programs as "This Is Your Life" and "Queen for a Day," in which essentially petty and prosaic tales of woe, perseverance, and triumph are accorded warm plaudits by studio audiences and handsome gifts by sponsors. It is difficult to imagine citizens of earlier or less affluent contemporary societies manifesting the same enthusiasm for such innocuous and inflated "life histories." See D. Riesman, *The Lonely Crowd, A Study of the Changing American Character,* New Haven: Yale University Press, 1950.

stay at a convalescent hospital, Norma returned home using crutches and wearing a full-length brace on her left leg, a pelvic band, and corrective shoes. There was a certain amount of residual weakness in her right leg as well, although not nearly so much as in the left. Norma needed her mother's help in bathing, dressing, and going to the toilet. She tired very easily and when tired made her way about in a wheelchair. Since stairs proved particularly difficult for her, the family installed a handrail along the stairway between the first and second floors of their home and at the front steps of the house. Despite these precautions, Norma frequently stumbled and fell during the first weeks at home. She was, of course, unable to engage in such pastimes as skating, jumping rope, hopscotch, and bicycle riding. Because of transportation and stair problems, Norma was unable to return to her old school, as she had fervently hoped to do; instead, she was registered in a special school for handicapped children.

Two months later Norma's condition showed only minor improvement. She stumbled less frequently and was able to handle her brace and crutches with more confidence. She used the wheelchair somewhat less often and did not tire quite so readily. But the primary functional incapacity remained. The family's hope that she would soon be fitted for a shorter brace had not been realized. Also, in the interim Norma had gained considerable weight, which caused added strain on her limited motor capacity. In this connection, Mrs. Mason said that she found it difficult to refuse Norma's requests for extra mealtime portions and between-meal snacks. Norma's annual summer visit to her grandmother was canceled because of her condition, and Mrs. Mason was hard pressed to find diversions for Norma that would keep her from becoming glum and despondent. Although on occasion the neighborhood children would still play with her, since it was summer, much of the time they were away on excursions of various kinds in which Norma could not join.

Four months later the doctor at the polio clinic recommended that Norma try to get about without her brace for part of the time. This experiment proved of limited success; she was able to move about the house by holding onto furniture and other objects, but she still had to use crutches outside her home. For distances of more than a city block or two, Norma had to put on the brace again, and she could not undertake longer excursions without auto transport. Norma could not easily use city busses, with their steep boarding platforms and narrow aisles, and she resorted to this means of transport only when accompanied by another person. Although there had been some improvement in the less affected right leg—she could lift it higher—in general, her functional state remained the same. In the meantime, Norma had returned to the school for handicapped children.

The following months witnessed no essential change in her over-all condition. The full-length brace remained, and the doctors said nothing about removing the pelvic band. Mrs. Mason abandoned the exercises recommended for Norma by the physiotherapist, because the girl seemed bored and the exercises "didn't seem to be doing any good anyway." After seeing on television the "true story" of a little girl who had had polio and grew up to become a swimming champion, Norma's mother enrolled her in a swimming class at the Y.W.C.A. This too was discontinued after several months, on the ground that the weather was too cold and Norma was subject to colds. Mrs. Mason talked of possibly sending Norma to the Polio Rehabilitation Center in Warm Springs, Georgia, where "they might be able to do something for her," but this proposal received no encouragement from the doctors or, for that matter, from Mr. Mason. He by this time was inclined to the view that the clinic at the convalescent hospital was doing as much as could be done for Norma.

When last seen, some fifteen months after Norma's discharge, the family seemed deeply discouraged over her condition. This was especially true of Mrs. Mason, despite her insistence that she had not given up hope that Norma would in time experience a fairly complete recovery. No improvement could be reported, however, except that Norma now managed to stoop on occasion, something she could not do previously. The child still used the same appliances and supports that she had used since discharge, albeit with greater skill and assurance. Shortly thereafter Norma returned to the hospital for surgery on her left ankle to try to correct a bad foot-drop.

For families like the Masons, in which the child remained functionally stationary, the recovery span of 12 to 18 months set forth by treatment personnel came to have a very different connotation than it did for families in the Progress Group. Once the reunion glow had faded, the child's apparent lack of progress imparted to this period the quality of a moratorium. Implicit in this perspective was the belief that the child, although he had not progressed until then, might well do so—and then perhaps with great rapidity—before time "ran out." Ten months after her daughter's discharge, or 17 months following onset, Mrs. Mason said: "From the very first they [treatment personnel] told me that there's no way of telling how far a muscle will come back. And since they explained it to me like that, I still have hope that she'll get a lot better than what she is."

Whereas Progress Group families converted the time span into something more structured and precise than it was meant to be, families in the Stationary Group made of it something more indefinite and occult. Both tendencies were attempts to sustain or generate hope, in the first case where reality appeared to confirm it, in the other where it seemed to be denied.

On occasion even the moratorium perspective assumed the superficial guise of a yardstick, as, for example, with Mrs. Paulus. Standing in great need of some tangible signs of progress because of the severity of her daughter's handicap, Mrs. Paulus tended to make much of such signs as a wiggle in Laura's toe, the occasional flicker of a calf muscle, and the 5-per-cent increase in muscle-strength rating given Laura at the last polio clinic. (There being a certain amount of variability in the physiotherapist's manual estimate of muscle strength from one occasion to the next, 5 per cent one way or the other is neither a meaningful nor a reliable figure.) Since Laura's over-all functional capacity did not improve over the entire period in which the family was seen, Mrs. Paulus' assiduous attention to minute and perhaps nonexistent changes appears to have been an attempt to transform psychologically the sterile moratorium situation into one pregnant with progress. If small gains can somehow be detected today, she seemed to be saying, greater gains are in store tomorrow.

In most of these seven families, it was only when time began to run out—roughly some twelve months following onset—that the moratorium mentality gave way to a more resigned sense of disappointment regarding the child's ultimate outcome. This was a long and slow process, full of vacillation, and in the year or so following discharge it was possible only to glean its beginnings. In none of the families was the process worked through to any marked degree. Perhaps it never is completely.

Typically, this process commenced with a tentative scaling down of hopes and expectations and an anticipatory consideration of negative possibilities. As progress failed to occur, the hoped-against possibility came to be imbued more and more with the character of an existential reality. The following statements by Mrs. Harris, in chronological order, illustrate this evolution toward resignation.

Two weeks following Marvin's discharge from the hospital:

Well, I think that Marvin will be all right. I mean, I think he'll help himself a lot to walk again. And they tell me that has a lot to do with it. You make up your mind that you're going to do something and you'll do it.

Two and a half months after discharge:

I have no idea [how Marvin will come along]. I mean, I just don't know. I know that my husband and I'll do everything we can—more than everything—to make him happy, and I think Marvin will walk some day without his brace. In my heart I know he will. And maybe once that hip gets enough strength in it, completely healed, that hip is going to help him to use the other parts of his leg better.

Four months:

I guess I don't expect anything for the two-year period. I mean, I feel like maybe he'll have to use the—[trails off]—the leg'll get a little stronger, then he could walk without the brace.

Eight months:

I don't know. I thought—I had more hopes. Now I don't know, I mean I thought that if it would improve a little bit more, it would have improved by now. I mean, it has been, you know, quite a while. And I thought there would be a little improvement, maybe a smaller brace or something. But I don't know. I mean, I hope that some day he won't have to wear the brace and he'll be all right, but I don't know. I mean I feel like that would be a big miracle.

Fifteen months:

Well, you know, the two years are almost up. So I guess we can't expect any improvement any more.

It is of interest that the physiotherapist who treated Marvin at the hospital told the interviewer at the time of Marvin's discharge that the boy's right leg was almost completely flail and that he would always require bracing, although subsequent corrective surgery might reduce somewhat the amount needed. The Harrises, however, became aware of this situation only gradually, and incompletely at that. This again indicates how treatment personnel sometimes infuse their prognoses with "uncertainty" for the purpose of "cooling the [family] out."

It would be misleading to assume that the expectational scaling-down process took place without interruption. Typically, the families in the Stationary Group vacillated between optimism and pessimism, hope and resignation, conviction and uncertainty. The felt unaccept-ability of a handicapped outcome, which they came increasingly to fear, characteristically induced a number of defense reactions that may in part be viewed as strategic for postponing, reducing, or re-defining the threat.

The most obvious of these reactions was to lengthen the period al-lotted for possible recovery beyond the 12 to 18 months posited by treatment personnel. In the statements quoted above, Mrs. Harris spoke repeatedly of "two years." The additional six months may represent her own rounding off of the time span or an "indulgence" from the doctor, who may have concluded that the Harrises were a "hard case" requiring more than the customary period in which to adjust psychologically to their child's handicap. An even more striking instance of this reaction is furnished by Mrs. Mason, who, on the basis of her misinterpretation of a statement made by Norma's physio-therapy teacher, remarked:

I'm still looking for improvement, and not exactly what the doctors told me about it taking only a year and a half to two years. The therapy teacher at Norma's school said she knows cases where they don't come along even after the year and a half or two years. And the way she talks, she thought it can happen in four to five years. I pray every night for that.

We have already touched on a second method of deriving and prolonging hope when the apparent condition of the child did not justify it. This was the tendency of some parents to resort, or to contemplate resorting, to channels of treatment other than those provided for or recommended by hospital treatment personnel. We have mentioned Mrs. Mason's television-inspired regime of swimming for Norma, and also her thoughts of sending the girl to Warm Springs. Similarly, the Mannings, as they grew more and more discouraged by Polly's lack of progress, began to consider borrowing money so that Mrs. Manning could take Polly to the Shrine of Lourdes in France. This, however, proved too costly an undertaking, and when last seen the Mannings had given up the plan in favor of a projected trip to the Shrine of Ste. Anne in Canada.

The greater frequency of prayers and the increased church attendance of several of the parents in the Stationary Group can also be regarded as a strategic appeal to other channels. It is significant to note that when last seen the Progress Group families had for the most part reverted to their old churchgoing habits: some went regularly; most, only occasionally; and a few, not at all. None, however, spoke any longer of feeling "closer to God" or realizing how important He was to them, as did several of the parents in the Stationary Group.

Finally—and this bears more on redefining the existing situation than on attempting to bring a more favorable one into being—there is the previously mentioned tendency to compare the child to someone worse off. In the Stationary Group families, this adoption of a negative point of reference became more and more prominent as the moratorium phase receded and the difficult psychic labor of devising long-range adjustments to the child's handicapped status began. The part played by the negative point of reference in this and subsequent developments can only be conjectured because the period during which the families were followed was not long enough for an established set of adjustments to have emerged. It would seem, though, that, in addition to the slight measure of consolation it may have afforded the family, this is a preferred, albeit not necessarily a satisfying, means for making the perceived downward transition from a more to a less favorable social identity.[3] By implication, this formula holds out two worlds, the better one that was and the worse one that could have been. Between these two worlds, the person who compares himself to someone less well off can begin to imagine his proper place, relate his past to his future, and articulate experimentally the host of meanings, images, and associations attendant on the status toward which he is evolving.[4]

THE FAMILY, THE DOCTOR, AND THE PHYSIOTHERAPIST

In the previous chapter we spoke of the important place physiotherapy came to occupy for the child and his family during the period of hospitalization—how it came to symbolize for them such key values as progress, will power, and purposive action. We also mentioned that the physiotherapist, in contrast to the doctors and nurses, frequently seemed to the family to be the only one who would take the trouble to "explain things" to them. Thus he won the position of a favorite hospital personage with many of the families. To these comments must be added the fact that the physiotherapist usually formed a very influential and close relationship with the child through his daily work of touching, holding, and manipulating the child's body—a degree of closeness that the average doctor could not begin to match with his occasional ward rounds and seemingly more impersonal approach.

The family's resulting confidence in the physiotherapist was generally of such a nature that they looked forward to additional and continuing benefits from physiotherapy after the child's discharge, particularly if the child returned home with more than a minor handicap. If physiotherapy could carry the child from an almost completely immobilized state to a point where he could ambulate on his own, could it not also carry him to a point where he could discard his brace or walk without a limp? So the parents reasoned.

[3] Similar rationalizations have been noted by students of the family during the depression. See E. W. Bakke, *Citizens Without Work*, New Haven: Yale University Press, 1940; and R. S. Cavan and K. H. Ranck, *The Family and the Depression*, Chicago: University of Chicago Press, 1938.

[4] See, in this connection, the illuminating discussion by Anselm Strauss of "Danger and Dispossession" in his *Mirrors and Masks*, Glencoe, Ill.: Free Press, 1959, pp. 36-39.

From a physiological standpoint, this question is more easily posed than answered, so variable are the determining factors from case to case. Doctors and physiotherapists in general agree that the amount of post-convalescent recovery that can occur through physiotherapy is inversely proportional to the amount of cellular destruction and resultant muscular incapacity wrought by the polio virus initially. Beyond this, however, they differ widely in emphasis.[5]

The doctor—in this instance an orthopedist—as a rule holds the view that once the post-acute phase of spontaneous recovery is over, only relatively limited functional advances can be gained through physiotherapy, particularly when muscles are moderately or severely denervated. The general tenor of the doctor's outlook can be inferred from the following statement:

> . . . It is futile to try to exercise muscles that are completely paralyzed or are so feeble that they have no functional value. It is futile and wasteful to continue with expensive physical therapy under these conditions. . . . The largest and most fruitful field of treatment of residual paralysis consists in the many orthopedic operations which have been devised to secure permanent correction of deformities and to improve the function of the extremities.[6]

With respect to the residual stage of the disease, therefore, the orthopedist usually thinks in terms of relatively fixed stages of motor capacity, which can be improved, if at all, most effectively and economically through corrective surgery.

The physiotherapist, by contrast, in many cases involving moderate to serious muscle incapacity, thinks more in terms of a gradual movement forward and an ongoing adjustment between potential and situation. Although he does not rule out either the possibility that corrective surgery will have beneficial effects or the possibility that an individual's residual paralysis can be so severe that a regime of physiotherapy will do him little good, he is more optimistic concerning the

[5] I am greatly indebted to Renée Fox for formulating and clarifying this issue for me. Also see N. Arnold, "The Adjustment of Adolescents to Poliomyelitis," *Journal of Pediatrics*, VL (September, 1954), 356-60.

[6] American Orthopaedic Association, "Infantile Paralysis, or Acute Poliomyelitis: A Brief Primer of the Disease and its Treatment," *Journal of the American Medical Association*, CXXI, (August 24, 1946), 1419.

potential benefits of a well-planned program of exercise and muscle re-education. Generally he leans to the view that weakened muscles, or muscles adjacent to the site of weakness, may, over a long period of time, be sufficiently enhanced in strength to substitute or compensate for a functional motor loss. Thus, although he does not promise a "cure"—and this, unfortunately, is not understood by many who place great hope in physiotherapy—he does as a rule hold that significant *rehabilitative* gains can frequently be brought about through physiotherapy, both prior to and following surgery, if surgery takes place.

We are not in a position here to judge the essential validity or relative merits of these two points of view.[7] But, in order to gain some understanding of the promise, problems, and performance of physiotherapy in the post-convalescent treatment of paralytic polio, we can at least compare what happened to those children among our 14 cases who continued to receive physiotherapeutic treatments following hospital discharge with what happened to those who did not.

Of the seven children who were discharged from the hospital in a seriously handicapped condition, arrangements were made in four cases (Paulus, Lawson, Manning, and Stewart) for a visiting physiotherapist to come to the home twice a week to treat the child. In another case (Mason), prior to the child's discharge the mother was instructed by the hospital physiotherapist on how to exercise the child. Later, as we have noted, this child also received some physiotherapy at a school for handicapped children. In the remaining two cases

---

[7] Although there are strong and conflicting opinions on this question, in our extensive review of the literature on polio rehabilitation, my colleagues and I failed to come across conclusive evidence on the matter. Quite apart, however, from whatever may be the intrinsic truth of its claims, there are important historical and sociological reasons for the adoption by the profession of physiotherapy of a distinctive point of view on this and related issues. To varying degrees, this derives from the marginal and poorly defined role of physiotherapy in many treatment centers; the changing pattern of recruitment to the profession (in recent years, an increasing proportion of men), and the gradual acceptance by the medical community of certain of Sister Kenny's views on the treatment of paralytic poliomyelitis. The last, in particular, appears to have significantly enhanced the role of the physiotherapist in polio rehabilitation. For an extended discussion of these matters see F. Davis, "Polio in the Family," unpublished doctoral dissertation, University of Chicago, 1958, pp. 146-48.

(Harris and Short), no physiotherapy was recommended at time of discharge, although Marvin Harris later received some at the same school for handicapped children attended by Norma Mason.

How much difference did post-hospital physiotherapy make in the cases of these children? It appears that some, by no means consistent, gains were made in the year or so following discharge. Of the six who received regular professional physiotherapeutic treatment during this period (including the two who, after some months, started physiotherapy at the school for handicapped children), only one, Johnny Lawson, progressed from a seriously to a moderately handicapped condition. (No doubt many orthopedists would maintain that owing to the nature of Johnny's residual incapacity this would have happened regardless of whether he had received any additional physiotherapy.) The other five, despite minor gains and improvements, remained seriously handicapped throughout this period. By contrast, the one seriously handicapped child who received no physiotherapy of any kind (Edward Short) did manage to progress to the moderately handicapped category.

These numbers are not very significant in themselves and prove nothing one way or the other about the efficacy of physiotherapy. I cite them only to point up the problems that confront the family—and the physiotherapist—when the post-hospital course of physiotherapy does not result in the kind and amount of progress hoped for and frequently expected. As in the early weeks of convalescence, when naïve optimism gave way to anxious pessimism, these families began to lose hope and wonder anew whether there was not some secret means by which they and the child could be brought back to the "normal" state of which they felt so bereft. They tended again to dwell on whether "all that could have been done had been done." Mr. Paulus, for example, said when last seen that had his daughter received hydrotherapy during her convalescence (a placebo-type treatment for the most part, according to treatment personnel) she would not, he believed, be so badly crippled. To the growing disillusionment with physiotherapy there was added in the meantime the continuing, and frequently heightened, dissatisfaction of the families with the scanty information given them by the hospital doctors when they brought the children in for periodic checkups at the polio clinic.[8]

Thus, for the parents of the more seriously handicapped children, it was as if they had come full circle: from the crisis-born faith in the great healing power of the modern doctor to the convalescence-inspired hope in physiotherapy back to the doctor—albeit at this later point they were considerably more disenchanted and ambivalently resigned to the "second best" promise of corrective surgery. But, to the extent to which the experience of these and other families appears to contradict the physiotherapist's claim that his knowledge and art can effect significant functional improvement in handicapped polio cases, several things must be said in his defense.

To begin with, while the child is still in the hospital, rarely does the physiotherapist feel that he is given sufficient time and professional assistance to work with the child as intensively as he would like. As in many specialized fields today, there is a dearth of trained practitioners. Furthermore, the chronic shortage of hospital beds may lead the physiotherapist to accede to discharging a child sooner than he would wish. Even more important, the sometimes unexpressed but always present desire of parents to have the child returned to them as soon as possible can be evaded and postponed for just so long. Although a convalescence of six months seems a very long time to the family, to the physiotherapist it is frequently barely long enough to make a start at rehabilitation.

Once the child has left the hospital and is out of his effective control, the difficulties, as the physiotherapist sees them, proliferate. A visiting arrangement is, he believes, a poor and uncertain substitute for daily ministrations carried out in his own domain. The family, he may state privately, is its own (and his) worst enemy as regards the effective implementation of a long-range program of home physiotherapy. The child is frequently allowed to become overweight; he is indulged when he should be disciplined; he is carelessly permitted to skip exercises or to do them only half-heartedly. In short, the family setting, with its many intangible and affectively loaded interpersonal

[8] Cf. Joseph Greenblum, "The Control of Sick Care Functions in the Hospitalization of a Child," *Journal of Health and Human Behavior*, II (Spring, 1961), 35.

ties, is, in his estimation, one of the worst possible ones in which to conduct the work of rehabilitation.[9]

Underlying all this there is the fundamental misconception held by many parents of what physiotherapy is and what it can accomplish. On this point, it may be said that the very success of physiotherapy during the first months of convalescence proves its later undoing. Witnessing the progress that the child makes in the hospital from bed to wheelchair to ambulation, and attributing this in large part to physiotherapy, the parents come to think of it as a "cure," a means of infusing life and motor force into damaged and destroyed muscles. This, as we have explained, does not and cannot happen. Physiotherapy—and, for that matter, any other form of medical treatment of residual polio paralysis—is a method of rehabilitation and not a cure. The paralysis must be accepted as given and efforts made to work around it or to compensate for it; it cannot be done away with.

For the families in this study, this understanding came slowly, incompletely, and in some instances not at all. In the previous chapter I discussed the various social and situational factors responsible for the failure of hospital personnel to communicate basic facts of the disease to the families during the period of hospitalization. These factors persisted for the most part through the course of post-convalescent physiotherapy at home. Again, the implied rationale for silence and evasion was that time would accomplish with less pain what words could accomplish, if at all, only with great distress and stark disillusionment to the hearer.

One may question whether the physiotherapist might not ultimately advance the cause of a long-range, conscientious acceptance of his

[9] Cf. T. Parsons and R. Fox, "Illness, Therapy and the Modern Urban American Family," *Journal of Social Issues*, VIII, 4(1952). This, of course, is the chronic complaint of the expert-specialist who, perhaps overvaluing the goals he holds out to his clients (as against the more general and intangible ones they hold out for themselves), often concludes that people are just too lazy, indifferent, or stupid to do what is in their own best interest. Perhaps it is incumbent on the physiotherapist, as on any number of other specialists, to take more considered account of how his scheme for betterment articulates with the numerous other demands, sentiments, and constraints impinging on the family. See Karl Mannheim, *Man and Society in an Age of Reconstruction*, New York: Harcourt, Brace, 1940, pp. 51-60; also Eliot Freidson, *Patients' Views of Medical Practice*, New York: Russell Sage Foundation, 1961, pp. 171-191.

regime by the family—and perhaps thereby better demonstrate what physiotherapy can accomplish—if, early in his contact with them, he carefully explained what rehabilitation as opposed to cure means, and how the distinction applies specifically to the child's condition. In doing so, he might also be performing a valuable social service for the family by directing some of its heavy emotional investment away from the unattainable "normal" state to one more realizable.

SOME IMPLICATIONS FOR REHABILITATION PHILOSOPHY

Because of his strategic role in rehabilitation, the foregoing remarks have focused mainly on the physiotherapist. It should be evident, however, that they have as much relevance for other treatment personnel (doctor, nurse, occupational therapist, hospital social worker) who are involved in mediating for the family information and attitudes about the disease and the condition of the child. In view of the complex division of labor among specialized health services in present-day hospitals and clinics, it would be unrealistic to expect the physiotherapist—or, for that matter, the doctor—to assume the whole of the considerable burden entailed in effecting a maximally therapeutic alignment of rehabilitational goals with family resources and expectations. All, to varying degrees, must contribute toward this end.

At the same time, it would be naïve to infer from the preceding pages that such an alignment would require only the frank and open communication of prognoses by treatment personnel to the family. Social-psychological research on a wide range of problems has shown that the communication of factual information in itself rarely changes attitudes, restructures expectations, or modifies social values. This is particularly true as regards issues that have high ego-saliency—i.e., in which the person has a deep emotional investment and about which strong social stereotypes that inhibit facile acceptance of new attitudes exist.

Clearly, a much more formidable task confronts rehabilitation workers if they are to impart to the family a truer and more balanced perspective of the child's illness and chances for recovery, if they are to guide them toward a more viable and ultimately less despairing means of adjusting to the child's impairment, and if they are to bring about a more enlightened appreciation of the potentialities, as well as the liabilities, of a physical handicap in our society. In addition to a more frank and full presentation of the facts, this kind of rehabilitational outlook would require treatment personnel to examine with family members what their feelings and attitudes are toward a "normal" as against a "less than normal" outcome. They would have to take up with the family the social and psychological, as well as physical, problems that are bound to affect the child and them. They would have to discuss and explore with them the merits and shortcomings of various schemes for coping with these problems.[10] Through such attempts to effect a more profound modification in the family's recovery perspective, the parent as much as the child would become the focus of therapeutic efforts.[11]

The ambitiousness of these aims cannot be gainsaid. But, in lieu of more enlightened and less prejudiced social attitudes toward the handicapped, they comprise the minimal demand that can legitimately be made of those to whom the handicapped turn for treatment and guidance. A physical handicap or chronic illness almost invariably involves changes in the whole life situation of the person, not just in his physical aspect. Rehabilitation must therefore be addressed to the whole breadth and complexity of the person's life situation so that his mind and body may be made to serve rather than nullify each other.

SUMMARY

Our major concern in this chapter has been the fate of recovery perspectives in the post-hospital period. Although all families experience a great burst of optimism upon the child's return home, in the ensuing months two distinctly different perspectives develop, depending mainly

[10] A discussion of how such programs might be implemented in polio convalescent centers as they are presently constituted would require a book in itself. Parent discussion groups, group psychotherapy, and role-playing immediately suggest themselves as some possible avenues along which such programs could be developed.

[11] H. B. Richardson, *Patients Have Families*, New York: Commonwealth Fund, 1946.

on the rate and amount of functional improvement demonstrated by the child in the home setting. In those families in which the child makes significant strides in his physical capacities (the Progress Group), an aura of achievement and a frequently unrealistic expectation of limitless improvement comes to characterize the outlook on recovery. For them, it is as if the child were exceeding some abstract yardstick of regularly scheduled increments of improvement.

By contrast, in those families in which the child shows little or no functional improvement (the Stationary Group), a moratorium psychology takes hold. The vague, overgeneral statement by doctors and others that improvement can occur within 18 months following onset of the disease is interpreted by the family to mean that if improvement has not already taken place it still might do so, all of a sudden and in one or two great bursts, "before the time runs out." It is only toward the end of this period, after still other rationalizations and reconstructions of "what the doctor meant" prove false, that the family seems prepared to accept a handicapped outcome for the child.

It is in the Stationary Group families especially that one sees the many deleterious effects resulting from the hospital's earlier failure to communicate prognoses and to grapple with the socio-emotional implications of crippling. These families continue to hope for a spontaneous "cure" long after the possibility has passed. Accordingly, opportunities for limited rehabilitative gains are neglected or, at best, only half-heartedly pursued.

Thus

Chapter 5. The Family: Role Performances and Relationships

far, our discussion has dealt mainly with issues directly related to the child's illness, its course and outcome. This, after all, constituted the locus around which the unique social and psychological situation of the family—e.g., hospitalization, separation, and recovery perspectives—came into being. In dealing with these matters, I have, perforce, portioned off but one large segment of the total life situation of the family—its immersion in and relationship to the special world of illness and the hospital—to the neglect, except incidentally, of other segments that have more to do with the effects of the experience on the family *qua* family. I refer to such questions as the functioning of the family during the child's absence and upon his return home, the effect of the experience on other members of the family, the various adjustments that the family attempts to make to the child's handicapped status—in short, how the family as an ongoing social entity, a unit that of necessity embraces matters both broader and more varied than those pertaining to the sick child alone, incorporates the polio experience into its life scheme.

In this chapter and in the one that follows, therefore, we shall view the family in its own setting, as distinct from that brought into being

by the hospital in connection with the child's illness. This is, however, not merely a matter of refocusing attention from one frame to
another. In turning away from the segmental and relatively clear lines
of the family-hospital relationship to the family alone, we become immersed in a complex setting in which cause and effect, motive and
act, purpose and consequence are linked in intricate, circular chains
through time and between persons. How, out of this simmering vessel
of primary social life, the place to which nearly all individual experience is "brought home" for synthesis and transmutation, can we
separate the influence of the illness experience from all else that has
transpired or is in the process of coming into being?

Consider, for example, the possible convergence of the illness-
associated problems in these 14 families with such commonplace
occurrences as the following: During the eighteen months or so in
which they were seen, five of the families moved to new neighborhoods,
one of them twice. Five of the fathers changed jobs, three of them
twice, and in most cases the job change was preceded by a period of
unemployment. Of the five job-changers, two changed occupations as
well. In one family, an older son married and left home. In two others,
the mother bore a new baby. Three of the polio children entered grade
school within a year after their discharge from the hospital. In four
families, illnesses or accidents of more than a minor nature occurred
involving one or both parents.

All these happenings, and countless others as well, had some direct
or indirect bearing on the problems posed by the child's illness and
physical disability. The presence in the family of a handicapped child
placed some fathers under greater compulsion to find a better paying
job. A mother incapacitated through illness became more than usually
upset by having to withdraw attention from the sick child. Change
of residence involved the handicapped child in the difficult task of
finding new neighborhood friends and playmates. Thus, matters that
at first seem remote from the crisis-engendered situation became en-
meshed with it and were soon modulated through the entire fabric of
family life and interrelationships.

Clearly, no single study can explore all these factors and their ramifications; ultimately some rather arbitrary limits must be set with
respect to the level and scope of analysis. Of the three main levels

at which the family has been studied by social scientists—as to its place and function in the larger society, as a culturally patterned set (or system) of interdependent roles, and as "a unity of interacting personalities"[1]—our discussion will focus mainly on the second. That is, I shall attempt to show how generalized family-member roles that are more or less common to all contemporary American families were affected by the long-term course of the illness experience.

In Chapter 2, we saw how the crisis elicits from family members certain pre-existent interactive roles that serve to channel and structure the experience. We noted that prior to the definitive diagnosis of polio, one parent, usually the mother, assumes the apprehensive role, while the other parent, usually the father, assumes the complementary role of comforter. In the more extended discussion of family roles that follows, I shall continue to use the concept "role" mainly in this interactional, rather than strictly structural, sense.[2] For apart from the new role of patient ascribed to the child by the hospital, and the segmental family-hospital roles brought into being by virtue of this, no new or additional positional roles accrue to family members as a result of the child's illness or, for that matter, his impairment when he returns home. What one witnesses, rather, are changes through time in the way in which family members perform their accustomed roles vis-à-vis the hospitalized and handicapped child. In some cases, as we shall see, such performances undergo marked change; in others, the alteration is relatively minor. But constituent intrafamilial structural roles remain fundamentally the same. The father, for example, retains his role of economic provider and final arbiter in matters of discipline; the mother retains hers of homemaker and attendant to the children's daily wants and needs; the children retain theirs as siblings and agents of parental goals and ideals.

[1] E. W. Burgess and H. J. Locke, *The Family,* New York: American Book, 1953.

[2] For a good discussion of these two uses of the role concept and their relationship to each other see Ralph H. Turner, "Role-Taking: Process *versus* Conformity," in Arnold M. Rose, ed., *Human Behavior and Social Processes,* Boston: Houghton, Mifflin, 1962, pp. 20 40. Useful conceptual distinctions among role, role prescription, role performance, and role behavior are also made by Robert F. Winch, *Identification and Its Familial Determinants,* Indianapolis, Ind.: Bobbs-Merrill, 1962, pp. 16-18.

By the foregoing, I wish to suggest neither that the family remains "basically the same" as a result of the experience nor that the changes in role performances occasioned by it are, in the short or long run, of no account. Even disregarding, as I have chosen to do, the more idiosyncratic personality and circumstantial factors that impinge on this situation from family to family, the typical changes in the performance of common family roles induced by the experience have significant effects on the equilibrium of family life. In this they engender a dynamic of their own that necessitates continual readjustment in the relationship of family members to one another. It is the characteristic vicissitudes of this process that I now wish to describe.[3]

THE FAMILY SETTING DURING THE PERIOD OF SEPARATION

The changes in family-member role performances induced by the child's illness and separation from home were fairly similar from family to family. In general, the members' appraisals of and behavior toward one another moved in the direction of greater leniency, indulgence, and concern. An air of greater tolerance and kind feeling infused the family atmosphere. Members—including sometimes even very young

[3] The descriptive account of this process that follows may, up to a point, usefully be conceived of in terms of Talcott Parsons' dynamic formulation of the phase movements of any social system (in this instance, the nuclear family) as it successively addresses itself to the ubiquitous functional problems of goal attainment, adaptation, integration, and tension management (or pattern maintenance). Here, we shall be concerned especially with phase movements of the family as it shifts its attention and effort between problems of integration and tension management. As we shall see, the peculiar integrative imbalances generated by the child's separation from home and subsequent reincorporation into it led to certain characteristic adjustments in the tension-management area. These, in turn, tended to aggravate integrational problems among family members and resulted in a refocusing of effort in this area.

In the following chapter, we shall be more concerned with the problem of the family's social-psychological adaptation to the external cultural environment as a result of the child's having been cast into a deviant social status, that of a visibly handicapped person. See T. Parsons, R. F. Bales, and E. A. Shils, *Working Papers in the Theory of Action*, Glencoe, Ill.: Free Press, 1953, pp. 163-269. A lucid account of the phase-movement formulation is to be found in E. C. Devereux, Jr., "Parsons' Sociological Theory," in Max Black, ed., *The Social Theories of Talcott Parsons*, Englewood Cliffs, N.J.: Prentice-Hall, 1961, pp. 53-63.

children—made fewer demands on one another, went out of their way more often for each other, and expected less of one another by way of fulfilling routine duties and tasks. This atmosphere persisted at least for the duration of the sick child's absence and usually for a period beyond as well, despite the many strains and difficulties it frequently generated.

Role-performance changes of this type embraced many facets of family life but were perhaps most evident in the area of child discipline. The invariable tendency among the parents was to shift away from policies of strictness, firm discipline, and "hardness" to greater permissiveness, indulgence, and "softness." Said Mrs. Eaton:

> I think, gee, I wish I hadn't done this to Geraldine, I wish I hadn't done that to Geraldine. And now what I'm afraid of is I'll start hollering, and I'll catch myself and think, now well maybe he [Geraldine's seven-year-old brother] could be in there [the hospital] too. And I'll catch myself that way. I don't fuss at them as much as I normally would have. But, I mean, I try to show more loving care for them.

Some parents stated that the distress of the sick child caused them to love and protect their other children all the more. Others expressed guilt for having been harsh with the sick child prior to his illness. Perceiving in the child's illness a kind of retribution for this "misdeed," such parents refrained from disciplining their other children in like fashion lest the same thing happen to them. For still other parents, the illness impressed upon them a sense of the frailty of childhood, and, for the time being at least, they found it convenient to hold that they "might just as well go easy with the children as be strict with them" because "you never know what's going to happen anyway." Whatever the reasons, however—although it should be pointed out that the themes of guilt and retribution figured prominently in this connection—a policy of leniency toward and indulgence of the children seemed to the parents the only just, logical, and appropriate one for the time and situation.

Naturally, the supreme object of the indulgence and concern of all other family members, in particular the parents, was the hospitalized child himself. Since he was situated for the time being outside the family setting and removed from its customary disciplinary controls, the parents had almost no other recourse but to heap special indulgences upon the child; all other relational modes were, given the situation, effectively closed to them. For example, even among the poorest families in the study, it was common for parents to initiate elaborate programs of gift-giving (e.g., a new set of toys every week), frequently far beyond the child's capacity to utilize the gifts and the parents' ability to afford them. Similarly, many of the mothers would sneak in favorite foods to the child on visiting days, a practice explicitly forbidden by hospital regulations. These tangible indulgences of the sick child, not to mention the many intangible emotional ones bestowed upon him, were justified typically by the parents as attempts "to keep his spirits up so that he'll have the will to get well."

Like the parents, the sibs of the hospitalized child felt pressures to respond to him with greater indulgence. Previous animosities, rivalries, and other expressions of sibling discord were at least temporarily laid aside and replaced by demonstrations of concern, affection, and sympathy for the sick child. (When as in some families a child of two or three seemed relatively oblivious of the plight of his sick brother or sister, his behavior was generally excused by the parents on the ground that "he's just too young to understand what's happened." The possibility that the barely socialized two- or three-year-old might have understood a great deal but reckoned it to his advantage to have his sib out of the house was apparently never entertained by the parents.)

Older children, however, were expected to, and apparently did, provide suitable behavioral testimony in behalf of the ill and absent sibling. According to the parents, they would inquire after each visiting day about the progress of their brother or sister, how much longer he would have to remain in the hospital, whether he would be able to play with them again, etc. Mrs. Eaton's description of her seven-year-old son's reaction to Geraldine's hospitalization is typical of those elicited from families in which there were other children of school age. (In an earlier interview Mrs. Eaton reported that Geraldine and her brother had fought constantly since early childhood and were forever complaining about each other.)

He's always asking me, "When's Gerry comin' home? . . . I sure wish she'd come on home." He makes all sorts of things at school for me to bring out to her when I visit. He didn't at first think about her being sick. He thought it was just something that everybody got and then got home soon. But now he realizes that she'll be in there for a while and he just wants her to get well and come home. That's all he talks about now.

In a few families, there seemed to be an almost defensive need on the part of the parents to portray the sib's involvement in his brother's or sister's illness in such terms as to leave little doubt that *everyone* in the family was "taking it hard." Mrs. Lee, for example, speaking of her older son Paul, said: "He thinks so much of his little brother Frankie that he told me he wished that he had gotten polio and been in the hospital instead of Frankie." (Paul, who was present when his mother made this remark, appeared to be embarrassed by it and left the room.)

In addition to these changes in family-member role performances there was, as we pointed out earlier, a rallying together of the neighborhood about the sick child and his family. The many expressions of sympathy, gifts, get-well cards, and offers of assistance all served to place the family "on stage," as it were. Even though other preoccupations and pursuits continued to engage them, they were constrained to enact their roles with that blend of sorrow, courage, altruism, and solidarity that American mores define as appropriate in such situations. Although several of the families might be regarded as deficient in one or more of these attributes, or inept in combining them harmoniously, the cultural image of the way in which a family should present itself in these circumstances appeared to exercise a strong influence on their self-appraisals and on what they told the interviewer.[4]

It is at least partially in this light that one must interpret the numerous reports by parents of increased family solidarity and intrafamilial amity as a result of the experience. Without doubt, such phenomena genuinely occurred to some degree in all the families, but not always,

[4] The most thorough discussion of these facets of public behavior is Erving Goffman, *The Presentation of Self in Everyday Life*, New York: Doubleday Anchor, 1959.

it would seem, to the degree reported. The Harris family affords a revealing, though perhaps somewhat extreme, case in point. In the first interview with the family, the parents remarked:

> *Mrs. Harris:* I'd say our marriage as far as being for each other, we always knew that we had a perfect marriage, only that we always seem to lack a little bit of money. That's all that I ever worried about. But starting this summer, having had it so bad [earlier that summer, before Marvin came down with polio, there had been a suicide in the family] I just felt like putting myself into a corner and staying there. And that kind of made my husband and me drift apart a little bit. Not that we loved each other less, but we just didn't talk or joke or have the happy life that we usually had. But with this happening [Marvin's polio], I guess we just wouldn't think of arguing or saying anything to each other, because we feel like nothing is important except Marvin.

> *Mr. Harris:* All those trivial things that we was arguing about aren't important.

But later in this interview and in subsequent ones, the mother, first subtly and later openly, complained of her husband's lack of success in his work and of his failure to support the family adequately. The picture of harmonious family relations was further belied by her complaints that close relatives and in-laws neglected and avoided the family, by reports of unusually selfish and demanding behavior on the part of the younger child during his sick brother's absence, and by further references to the inadequacies of her husband as a breadwinner. In this family, and in several others as well, the statements about greater solidarity and amity had relevance primarily at the testimonial level.

But even granting the emergence of a higher degree of solidarity during the period of the child's absence, strains and tensions soon became evident in the functioning of most of the families. I shall discuss the most typical of these here, disregarding the by no means unimportant problems that were of a more circumstantial and adaptive character—e.g., the mother's having to alter her daily routine and arrange for baby sitters while she visited the sick child at the hospital, the father's having to seek special permission from his employer to take time off during working hours to visit the child.

As a result of the sick child's absence from home and the more lenient attitudes adopted toward the other children, the remaining children, according to many of the parents, soon became more "spoiled," "pampered," and "too much the center of attention around here." Disciplinary practices were upset and came to deviate markedly from established patterns. For example, Mrs. Johnson, whose husband felt guilty over having beaten his son with a strap several days before the boy was taken to the hospital, complained that Mr. Johnson never spanked the other children "since Dickie went up there." Because of this, she claimed, the enforcement of discipline had fallen wholly on her shoulders, with the result that the three remaining children accused her of being harsher and more severe with them than she basically was or wished to be.

Parental relations with the hospitalized child also gave rise to numerous problems. In Chapter 3 we discussed the loosening of the sick child's affective ties with home and the variety of ways in which the hospital accomplished this. From the parents' standpoint, the danger was that the child would become oversocialized to the hospital to the detriment of his ties with home. Evidences of this fear, in varying degrees and in different ways, appeared in nine of the families, and in several of them it clearly became a matter of considerable concern. Mrs. Richards, for example, reported sorrowfully after Neil had been in the hospital for four months: "Neil seems to be growing away from us. Seems more like he belongs to the hospital."

As discharge time approached, several of the children were reluctant to leave the hospital, usually attributing their wish to remain to forthcoming parties and other entertainments that the hospital had scheduled for Halloween, Christmas, or Easter. One twelve-year-old stated defiantly that she could have much more fun in the hospital at Christmas than she could at home, and that she did not want to leave before then. A seven-year-old boy whose family was the poorest of the fourteen had virtually to be dragged away from the hospital, and for days thereafter he cried incessantly and insisted that he wanted to return. Incidents of this kind naturally troubled the parents, especially since they had taken great pains to be extra-indulgent of the hospitalized child. Although they never said as much, it is easy to surmise that the child's ambivalence about returning home led them to conjecture uneasily about their adequacy as parents.

Usually, however, strains involving the nonmedical side of hospitalization developed around the question of supplying the sick child with a steady stream of gifts and toys, which nearly all the children came to expect and demand as a matter of course. This situation was aggravated by the child's observation of other children on the ward receiving many gifts and his natural wish to be treated similarly. Not only did this make for a significant financial drain on the family—seeing what was going on, the sibs of the sick child also demanded, and usually received, equal treatment—but, more important, many of the parents began to feel that the sick child was becoming much too spoiled and demanding as a result of hospitalization and that these changes in his character would persist and make him more difficult to get along with once he returned home.[5] As Mrs. Eaton said of her daughter Geraldine:

> I'm afraid she's getting awfully spoiled in the hospital with all the attention and presents people have been giving her. Every time I see her she just hands me a list of things she wants me to bring her the next visiting day, and she usually gets them too. I say, it's like Christmas! I just hope she doesn't expect the same thing when she gets home.

In general, hospitalization raised delicate and precarious issues for the family. The young child was expected somehow to demonstrate an emotionally appropriate division of loyalties and attachments between home and hospital. This subtle task, as I have indicated, frequently exceeded the discriminatory capacity that his level of maturation permitted.[6] The parents, on their part, found themselves under considerable internal and external pressure to adopt more lenient and indulgent attitudes toward him, and often toward the other children

[5] The failure of doctors and others to take into account these effects of long-term hospital confinement on children is discussed insightfully by Sir J. C. Spence, *The Case of Children in Hospitals,* lecture delivered at the Royal College of Physicians, London, November 19, 1946. Reprinted by the Federal Security Agency, Social Security Administration, Washington 25, D.C.

[6] A revealing and amusing incident to this effect was reported by Mrs. Lawson. After she and her husband had spoken at length with their eight-year-old son about how important it was for him to learn to like the hospital, to cooperate with the doctors and nurses, etc., he remained silent for a few moments and, on the verge of tears, asked, "Is it all right for me to feel a little homesick too?"

as well. This, in turn, produced other imbalances within the family setting, along with some apprehension over the post-hospital behavior and character of the absent child. Also, hospitalization, while it seldom results in a total cessation of normal childhood socialization, does, at minimum, represent a significant diversion thereof. This, as we shall show in the section to follow, had characteristic consequences for interaction and relationships in the family once the child returned home.

Generalizing on these role-performance changes in the family during the first months, it can be said that the illness and removal of the sick child from home resulted in heightened attentiveness of family members to one another's ego-supportive needs.[7] This, in turn, engendered numerous strains and difficulties in the enactment of conventional, mutually regulatory social-control roles in the family and in the maintenance of the norms that sustain them.

THE FAMILY SETTING WITH THE CHILD RETURNED: SOURCES OF DISEQUILIBRIUM

The changes in family-member role performances during the period of hospitalization constituted the framework for the series of adjustments that the family had to make once the child returned home. Characteristically, his return occasioned in the family what may be termed a state of socio-political imbalance, especially as regards the nature and exercise of parental authority and the behavioral norms that govern sibling relations. The absence of the sick child from the family circle had permitted the parents to pursue different, and often contradictory, policies toward him and his siblings. The temporal and spatially separate backgrounds of these family transactions (home and hospital) permitted such inconsistency, an anomaly that even the parents themselves seemed to recognize. The child's return, however, brought these matters sharply into simultaneous focus, and the inevitable result was conflict, indecisiveness, and a host of ambiguities as

---

[7] Cf. Talcott Parsons, "Definitions of Health and Illness in the Light of American Values and Social Structure," in E. Gartley Jaco, ed., *Patients, Physicians and Illness*, Glencoe, Ill.: Free Press, 1958, p. 185.

the family sought somehow to stabilize its functioning at a workable level.

Conflict, indecisiveness, and inconsistency arose mainly from three sources: (1) the difficulty of abandoning the parental policy of greater leniency and indulgence toward the children that, for the sick child, at least, continued unabated throughout his hospital stay and could not be altered immediately upon his return; (2) the behavioral and, in some cases, seemingly characterological changes induced in the sick child as a result of his hospital experience; and (3) the uncertainty and ambivalence of parents concerning the proper handling of the returned child in view of his hospital experience and his residual impairment.

The Problem of Altering Styles of Parental Authority

The first of these points has already been touched on. Little need be added here, save that the crisis-provoked pattern of indulgence of the sick child invariably carried over into the period of reunion glow. Much as they might have wished or thought it advisable to do so, the parents could not immediately upon the child's return abandon the many kindnesses and special indulgences that for months past they had lavished upon him. As in all such continuing relationships, this facet of their behavior toward the child had to be phased out gradually while other, less one-sided controls in the reward-punishment balance slowly made themselves felt.[8]

Had this factor been the only obstacle to the resumption of smooth family functioning, the task would have been an easy one. Deeper and more pervasive disturbances, however, were occasioned by the child's return.

Hospital-Induced Behavioral Changes in the Child

Behavioral changes growing out of hospitalization were evident in all the returned children, although the degree and duration of such changes varied from child to child. Typically, following his homecoming the child was described by his parents as being in some ways "more grown up," "more mature," "more of a man," "more ladylike,"

[8] See Anselm Strauss, *Mirrors and Masks,* Glencoe, Ill.: Free Press, 1959, pp. 124-31.

etc., than before, while in other ways he was described as "more spoiled," "too demanding," "possessive," "selfish," or "too aggressive." The apparent contradiction implied in these descriptions can perhaps be understood if we consider the kind of socialization that the average child undergoes in a hospital as contrasted with what he ordinarily experiences at home.[9]

In the hospital, certain facets of that complex body of learning we call childhood socialization are accelerated, while others are retarded or inhibited. The relations of the hospitalized child to the authority figures who attend to him are, on the whole, clearly delineated and segmental in character. A mechanical egalitarianism prevails among the children. For purposes of maintaining control and for the administrative convenience of staff, one child on the hospital ward is treated very much like the others; his privileges and punishments are meted out according to a largely impersonal code which, to a much greater extent than can ever be true in the home, focuses on his present person to the relative neglect of his past and future persons.

In this milieu, the child soon acquires a relatively simple and mechanical understanding of *his* rights, duties, and privileges and of the parallel rights, duties, and privileges of the other children on the ward. Since the child has no familial or other enduring ties with his wardmates or staff, he finds it expedient to treat his toys, comic books, and other prized possessions as belonging clearly to him and to no one else. Besides, were such rights of possession permitted to become blurred, as they constantly are in the family setting, the nurse would soon become involved in the delicate task of adjudicating ownership according to criteria that are less orderly, impersonal, and mechanical than those which she customarily employs. This, of course, would also tend to distort the neat lines of authority that radiate symmetrically from her to every child on the ward.

These qualities of life on the ward as perceived by the child are suggested in the "list of rules" that Johnny Lawson and several of his wardmates drew up for membership in their "club." The document, a penciled affair of elaborate marginal design, was given by

[9] Cf. Joseph Greenblum, "The Control of Sick Care Functions in the Hospitalization of a Child," *Journal of Health and Human Behavior*, II, 1 (Spring, 1961), 37-38.

Johnny to the ward nurse, who in turn showed it to the Project's psychologist:

HILLSIDE HOSPITAL CLUB

Good Chart

1. Do not talk at nap
2. Do not talk at dinner
3. Do not talk at night
4. Do not be bad
5. Do not talk in school
6. Be a good sport
7. Do not shoot sticks
8. Do your homework when the teacher tells you to
9. Do not say bad words
10. Do not swear
11. Do not talk so loud
12. No toys on bed pan
13. Obey the nurses
14. Listen to the doctors
15. Little folks should be seen and not heard
16. Do not fight or throw things
17. Kiss the girls all you want
18. Do not trade toys
19. Don't throw toys
20. Be good at the workshop

In a certain sense, the attitudes of compliance toward a relatively impersonal institutional authority that come to be instilled in the hospitalized child bear at least a superficial resemblance to the social forms by which an adult is expected to conduct himself in civil society. In the hospital, the child learns to say "please" and "thank you" at the appropriate times. The shyness and drawing away that so often overcome him in the presence of strangers are to a certain extent dispelled as a result of the ample practice afforded him in conducting relatively impersonal relations with doctors, nurses, and others who daily attend to him. He becomes socially more at ease, so to speak. Apparently it was primarily this kind of behavioral change in the returned child that led the parents to describe him as "more grown up," "more mature," "less babyish," and the like.

But, just as this facet of the child's socialization is accelerated in the hospital, so are others retarded, inhibited, or allowed to remain dormant. The same set of structural relations that, on the one hand, encourages sociability fosters, on the other hand, greater possessiveness, competitiveness, and, in general, a less flexible sense of ego boundaries. Returned to the family setting, with its diffuse role relationships and its less punctilious styles of authority, the child frequently finds it difficult at first to behave in a "brotherly" or "sisterly" fashion toward the other children in the family. For a time at least, he is likely to act toward them in accordance with the crude egalitarian norms that governed his relationships in the hospital. This frequently appears to parents as self-centeredness and—as is so often true of persons who reside in institutions and become practiced in covert rule evasion[10]—as evidence of a too keen appreciation of immediate advantage to be grasped whenever authority is not looking.

In summary, the lengthy hospital confinement of the children generally caused them to regress somewhat with respect to what might be termed the de-egocentrizing goals of childhood socialization, from what for most of them was a rudimentary capacity to internalize superego controls to an earlier stage of psycho-social development in which such controls are largely external in nature. Concurrently—as we shall soon see—this also contributed significantly to the problem of role-performance integration in the family.

Over the long term, however, the permanence and seriousness of such disruptions in the course of normal childhood socialization appear to depend mainly on their congruence with continuing, more pervasive patterns of interpersonal relations in the family. Thus, for example, a strong pattern of sibling rivalry or some gross asymmetry in the parents' emotional orientation toward the children (e.g., mother always punishing, forbidding, and quarrelsome and father always indulgent, easygoing, and lax) seemed to prolong the child's hospital-altered behavior for a longer period than was the case in families in which such patterns were absent or less marked.[11] In at least seven

---

[10] See Erving Goffman, *Asylums, Essays on the Social Situation of Mental Patients and Other Inmates,* New York: Doubleday Anchor, 1961, pp. 189-93.

[11] Cf. Philip E. Slater, "Parental Role Differentiation," *American Journal of Sociology,* LXVII, 3 (November, 1961), 296-308.

of the families (including some in which the child remained significantly handicapped as well as some in which he did not) its effects could be seen for as much as a year after his return home. But, in the first months following his return, the unanimity with which parents reported the child's behavior as "more selfish," "uncooperative," "demanding," and "possessive" was striking.

Ambivalent Identification of the Handicapped Child

Allied with hospital-induced behavioral changes in the child and aggravating the problem of his discipline was parental uncertainty about how to treat him because of his having had polio, his having been away from home, and, most important, his being handicapped. This became the major adjustment problem in the nine families in which the child remained handicapped to some significant extent. In the five in which the child recovered to a point at which his handicap was minimal or nonexistent, the problem eventually became much less an issue, although even here vestigial traces of it could be detected for some time. In either case, the full significance of this factor for the life of the family is of such overriding social-psychological interest that I have chosen to deal with its many ramifications in a separate chapter (Chapter 6). Suffice it to indicate here that, as regards the disciplining of the returned child, the parents were confronted in essence with a situation of marginal identification. In innumerable respects the returned child was the same child he was before his illness; yet in several crucial and dramatic respects he was greatly changed. This mixed and vacillating perception of the child tended to throw into question for the parents customary modes by which they disciplined him.

CONSEQUENCES FOR CHILDHOOD SOCIALIZATION PRACTICES

The varied effects emanating from this constellation of factors making for disequilibrium can perhaps best be seen in the context of certain basic modalities of childhood socialization in our society: (1) reward-punishment, (2) dependence-independence, and (3) equality-differentiation in sibling roles. Although for purposes of discussion these are phrased as polar dichotomies, it should be understood that what transpired in the families was not the supplanting of one extreme attribute by its polar opposite. The typical occurrence, rather, was a shifting and realignment of valences away from one end *toward* another. Each family, however, revealed its own distinct cluster of starting points and end states, so to speak, across these dimensions of socialization.

Reward-Punishment

The socialization of any child, regardless how permissive or harsh the parents are, involves the application of some relatively stable balance of rewards and punishments in his discipline. As is true of families in general in our society, the families in the study differed greatly in their methods of rewarding and punishing their children. Some parents appeared to be quite strict; others were very lenient. Some, when their children misbehaved, typically resorted to corporal punishment or angry vocal assaults; others employed deprivational measures, such as making the child sit in a corner, sending him off to his room, or withdrawing his television-viewing privilege.

Regardless of the particular balance or style of rewards and punishments that had been employed by the parents prior to the child's illness, he was invariably subjected to a different pattern of discipline following his return from the hospital. This always tended in the direction of less frequent and less severe forms of punishment, greater toleration for a wider range of misbehaviors, and, in general, a more indulgent and compromising response to the child's conduct. Said Mr. Paulus:

> I'd say I give in to her a lot more than I used to. Like the other night she said she wanted to go see this here Walt Disney movie down at the Orpheum. Well, I took her to see it the very next night. But figuring ordinarily, if Laura hadn't been sick I might not have jumped right up like that. But, I mean, I feel that if there's something nice that children can do and she can do too, like that movie, I like to help her out with it.

Especially during the first months following the child's return though in several of the families, for long thereafter—this leniency and reluctance to administer usual forms of punishment was as pronounced among the parents of the minimally handicapped children as it was among those whose children were seriously handicapped.

Independence–Dependence

In a broad and general sense, socialization can be thought of as the history of the person's evolution from dependence to independence through the stages of infancy, childhood, adolescence, and young adulthood. It is of the very essence of this developmental process that, with increasing age, the person's status in the family and in society changes. Actions that formerly required the consent, approval, and guidance of others are replaced gradually, though sometimes abruptly, by others that are more or less self-initiated and self-accountable.

In the 14 families this rarely smooth process became a focal point for seemingly greater than usual strain, conflict, and emotional complexity. Parents feared that if they allowed the returned child as much freedom as they had prior to his illness, he could easily do injury to himself because of his impairment and residual weakness. In many instances they also "felt sorry" for him and wished through special care and treatment somehow to "make it up to him." In general, then, they tended to be more protective of the child and tried to help him much more than they would ordinarily have done. At the same time, however, the parents were concerned lest this "spoil the child," making him *too* dependent on them. They feared that such overdependence might prevent the child from growing into a "real man" or "real woman." Periodically, therefore, they would reproach themselves for having been too helpful and too indulgent and would vow to let the child "do things for himself" in the future.

The returned child, particularly if he was very young (e.g., five to seven) or not too severely handicapped, could not always appreciate his parents' efforts to be more protective, much less their attempts to restrict him to certain activities. Usually he felt under some compulsion to prove that he was "no different from" and "just as good as" other children, and that his inability to participate fully in play and games was just a temporary state of affairs. His constant testing of this proposition often resulted in frustration and unhappiness as well as in scolding by the parents. Frequently projecting the cause of his failure onto his parents, he would reverse his attitude—just as they periodically did theirs—and demand from them extra attentions and indulgences by way of compensation. The parents, as a rule—perhaps acting out of guilt, pity, or the sheer fatigue brought on by too much turmoil—seemed more than willing to supply these extras.

The effect of such volatile interaction was a heightened ambivalence and confusion on the part of both parents and child as to which activities called for greater dependence and which for less. The never very explicit guides on which contemporary American parents rely in these matters seemed to these families even vaguer and more equivocal than they do ordinarily. The following reports give some indication of the confusion and ambivalence parents experienced:

> *Mrs. Manning:* Once in a while she'll say to me, "Why don't you let me go out?" And I'll say, "Well, go ahead. Go out and play if you want to." Then she gets a little downhearted and she'll say, "Oh, I don't want to play. I want to do something else." She'll think of something else to do. And I try to explain to her that she just has to do things that don't take so much energy.

> *Mrs. Harris:* It seemed when Marvin returned home like everything I did for him just wasn't good enough, and it made me feel bad. I think that was just the first week of being home. . . . I mean I don't want him to be spoiled, and if he does something I'll holler at him. And—but he just hollers right back. You know, he's not a baby any more. He's a big boy.

As the foregoing quotations suggest, "double-bind" phenomena of the type described by Bateson and his colleagues[12] proliferated in these families: viz., the parents often verbally supported the child's attempts to do as other children did while at the same time emotionally discouraging these attempts by holding out affectional rewards for non-performance. Independent action therefore became a source of anxiety for the child, with performance symbolizing covert parental disapproval and probable failure and non-performance symbolizing reward and safety, but ego degradation as well. Both alternatives were unsatisfactory, and regardless of which was chosen there followed a

[12] G. Bateson, D. Jackson, J. Haley, and J. Weakland, "Toward a Theory of Schizophrenia," *Behavioral Science,* I (October, 1956), 253-56.

chain of emotionally charged incidents that aggravated the underlying conflict and ensnared both parent and child more tightly in the trap of their ambivalences.[13]

Equality—Differentiation in Sibling Roles

It was in the area of sibling relations that family disturbances were most evident and widespread following the child's homecoming. Beyond certain customary differences in the patterning of age-sex roles of siblings (although these too are less sharply differentiated in the contemporary American family than formerly), the American family more nearly approaches perfect egalitarianism in the realm of child rearing than does the family in any other Western or Western-influenced society. Without considering here the many intrapsychic and societal implications of this statement, it can easily be surmised how the situation of the returned child challenged various norms of sibling equality and made it difficult to realize them in daily family life.[14] As I have pointed out, not only did the returned child frequently expect preferential treatment, but the parents were often inclined—albeit sometimes ambivalently—to accord it to him.

In the nine families in which the returned child had one or more sibs close to him in age, there occurred a natural history of appeasement, conflict, and resolution. During the early post-discharge stage, the sibs of the returned child, usually in response to parental coaxing and admonitions, treated him in an indulgent manner, performing special favors for him, freely letting him play with their toys, and even at times appearing to rejoice in the special place accorded him in the family circle. It was not unusual at this stage for a sib to accom-

[13] See the discussion of the Harris family, pp. 152-57.

[14] See, for example, Burgess and Locke, *op. cit.*, and M. Mead and M. Wolfenstein, *Childhood in Contemporary Cultures,* Chicago: University of Chicago Press, 1955. This, of course, is not to suggest that the American parent feels exactly the same about all his children, never subjectively favoring one child over another. Rather, the generalization points to the policy aspect of child rearing: i.e., the parents' moral conviction that, within broad limits, there should be equality of treatment of the children, regardless how they may feel subjectively about their several charges. That there often is a discrepancy between policy and its execution goes without saying. This, however, is no reason for viewing the policy dimension as unimportant or merely incidental, a tendency too often found in psychological and psychoanalytic analyses of family relationships.

pany the handicapped child wherever he could not go on his own and to act as his constant companion and helper.

This stage of appeasement sooner or later gave way to the conflict stage, in which the sib renounced his unaccustomed stance of benevolence and expressed resentment to his parents over the one-sided nature of his relationship with the polio child. He would decry the inequities that he felt were being perpetrated by the parents and would often strike back at the polio child. As Dick Johnson's younger brother Kenneth was reported to have told him prior to punching him: "I don't care if you do have polio, I'm going to fight you anyway."

The turmoil and strife of this stage invariably led the parents, and sometimes the children themselves, to adopt a new *modus vivendi* in sib relations. Although this seldom took the same form as existed prior to the sick child's illness, the imbalance was usually redressed to a certain extent, with more or less exclusive compensations and privileges being accorded each child. This process was most dramatically illustrated in the Prince family, which consisted of the parents, five-and-a-half-year-old David, the polio child, and nine-and-a-half-year-old Harold.

Before David's illness, he had always been the aggressive one and the instigator of fights with his brother. After futile attempts to shrug off David's attacks, Harold's temper would reach the breaking point and he would use his greater height and weight to smack David down. This scheme of things had come to be accepted, more or less, by the parents as both natural and proper.

During the time David was in the hospital, however, Harold—a somewhat conscience-ridden youth—fervently vowed that when David returned home he would be "the best brother in the world to him," would keep him out of trouble, and would even do David's physiotherapy exercises with him. The parents were pleased by these expressions of fraternal devotion but unconvinced of Harold's ability to restrain himself when provoked. Hence, they did not refrain from warning him, before David's homecoming, that if he "so much as laid a hand" on his sick brother, he would "really catch it." Harold assured them that the days of fighting and ill will between David and himself were over.

Unfortunately, upon his return home David was not of a similar turn of mind. Quite the contrary; his pre-polio aggressiveness seemed aggravated. He appropriated many of Harold's playthings and refused to share any of the vast number of toys he had received during his hospital stay. For a time following his homecoming, David was a veritable *enfant terrible*, intimidating the family with inconsolable temper tantrums. For example, Mrs. Prince, contrary to Jewish practice, was forced to violate the traditional Passover prohibition of serving leavened bread because David insisted on being served toast every morning, Passover or no Passover.

Needless to say, relations between the brothers soon deteriorated, and one day, frustrated beyond endurance, Harold did "lay a hand" on David. As warned, he "really caught it" from his father, who promised an even more severe beating if he struck his younger brother again. Following this, Harold began to complain of a series of vague ailments suggestive of psychosomatic origin—headaches, backaches, pains in the legs. Mrs. Prince finally took him to the family doctor who, after examining Harold and speaking with him privately for several minutes, reprimanded her for not allowing Harold greater freedom, losing her temper with him too easily, and placing too little trust in him.

In the succeeding months, this lecture and the parents' growing conviction that David was "having his own way too much," often at Harold's expense, led to certain changes in the family. Harold was again permitted to strike David when he was justifiably angry, but only "lightly" and "never on the legs." David's discipline was as much as possible turned over to Mr. Prince, who seemed somewhat more adept than his wife at keeping the boy in check. The parents were finally able to put an end to the toy-a-week policy that had continued long after David's return home, much to the resentment of Harold, who was not similarly indulged.

SUMMARY AND IMPLICATIONS

In the preceding pages I have described what occurred in the families with respect to certain key aspects of childhood socialization. Other areas of family life might have been chosen as well to illustrate the changes and stresses experienced in the wake of the child's hospitalization and homecoming. To have done so, however, would have made for greater descriptive diffuseness in that, what little else the families may have shared by way of circumstances, setting, and interactional style of life, all at least were involved in the usually consuming task of raising children.

Even though limited to this facet of family life, the discussion has been extremely general because of the distinctive issues and interpersonal themes among the families and the sometimes idiosyncratic interplay of these with the illness experience as such.[15] Yet, at a more abstract level of analysis, all the families can be thought of as having undergone the same process of readjustment: with the return of the child, the shifts and re-emphases in family-member role performances occasioned by the child's illness and hospitalization engendered certain characteristic imbalances in the family's functioning. These imbalances, in turn, led to still other adaptations and accommodations within the family setting.

The foregoing is, I realize, little more than a reiteration of the familiar dynamic of the family adjustment process, one that applies to other family crises as well as to this one and, for that matter, to much of the ordinary give-and-take of family life. Indeed, if we allow ourselves to overlook the vast reservoir of intimate and individuated experience that forms so distinctive a part of family life and instead treat the family as but another kind of social system, we can, with Parsons[16] and others, discern much in this process that corresponds with the phases and cycles through which any organization passes as it routinely attempts to balance the internal and external demands made upon it. In the instance examined here, the functional disturbance was of more than routine dimensions. Hence, more than normal effort had to be expended to keep the system functioning.

For the sociologist, such expenditures have the virtue of making the "machinery" of the ongoing adjustment process more visible, thereby bringing to light conditions, connections, and consequences that might

[15] A most sensitive analysis of distinctive psycho-social themes in a cross-section of normal families is Robert D. Hess and Gerald Handel, *Family Worlds*, Chicago: University of Chicago Press, 1959.

[16] Parsons, Bales, and Shils, *op. cit.*

otherwise remain obscure or problematical. Thus, in the preceding pages, we were able to show the extremely close and mutually dependent interplay in the family of phase adjustments in the areas of tension-management and role-performance integration. It remains for future research to determine whether there is something unique about the contemporary urban family that subjects it to a high degree of phasic interdependence in these areas, or whether it shares this characteristic to approximately the same extent with other social organizations. As our knowledge on these questions increases, we may discover that, whereas all social systems must at one point or another be concerned with essentially the same four problems of equilibrium maintenance,[17] the particular phase sequences that emerge in the process of making these adjustments differ from one system to the next, depending on the system's primary purposes, structure, and location in some larger social order.

As for the nature, scope, and duration of the illness-generated adjustment process in these particular families (as distinct from its content in any given family), certain tentative conclusions can be advanced on the basis of our data.

First, the process proved on the whole much more difficult, prolonged, and pervasive in those families in which the child remained handicapped to some significant extent than it did in those families in which he did not. Among the latter, such illness-associated disturbances as could still be detected in the family eighteen months later had become almost indistinguishable from the family's historical pattern of interaction and relationships. By contrast, among the former families, the disturbances—while by no means divorced from primary intrafamilial processes—maintained themselves with a kind of self-generating potential, forever giving rise to new compromises and adjustments. In no meaningful sense can it be said of the families in which the child remained handicapped that the problems and conflicts arising from his situation had been resolved, much less solved, during the period of the study. An accomplishment of this magnitude would have been virtually impossible, if only because the handicapped child was approaching, or had yet to approach, age and peer statuses in

[17] *Ibid.*

which his impairment was to acquire new and usually more profound significance. Thus, for example, many of the parents in this group saw their major problem, not as a present one, but as one in the easily forseeable future—"when he gets older and starts noticing girls," "when all her friends begin dating and go off to dances," "when he's a teen-ager."

Secondly, where the illness-associated problems persisted for a long period of time, there appeared to be a tendency for them to merge with older and continuing issues of tension and conflict in the family. Several illustrations of this were given in the body of the chapter. Here we might note further that the joining of the new problem with the old served, for a time at least, to exaggerate the old tensions and conflicts.[18] This often had the effect of masking from family members certain unique features of the new difficulty (e.g., their negative or ambivalent feelings toward the child's handicap) while simultaneously generating strong pressures for a resolution of what was thought to be essentially "the same old problem" several times magnified. Characteristically, the attempts that followed failed, if only because they did not take adequate account of what was new and different in the family's situation.

Such failures, though, were but the inverted representation of what, from another vantage point, could be regarded as strength and continuity in these families. For, despite the many stresses and disturbances occasioned by the child's illness and disability, none of the families showed anything approaching a profound alteration in its underlying scheme of life, or in its understanding of the scheme's meaning, design, and purposes. Much less can it be said of them that they were "disorganized" by the experience. On the contrary, one sensed in these families a persistent and almost tenacious sameness; a sameness that in the very midst of surrounding changes imparted to each day, week, and month much the same tone, pace, and quality of being as the one preceding and the one following. This might simply be the outward manifestation of a deeply ingrained, self-protective unaware-

---

[18] A worthwhile subject for further research would be to determine the extent to which a range of externally induced stresses on the family are reduced, merged, and synthesized with pre-existent and pervasive forms of conflict within it.

ness. Conversely, or perhaps concomitantly, it might bespeak a fundamental stability in the family, enabling it with reasonable facility to absorb the impact of the polio experience while at the same time insulating it from both serious disorganization and creative reorganization. As is so common in social life, what constituted strength in these families was also, as we shall see, a major source of weakness.

THROUGHOUT

Chapter 6. The Family:
Some Problems of Identity

this work we have frequently pointed to some of the problems of identity and self-image confronting the sick child and his family. Thus, in the discussion of the crisis period, we saw how the family, when it was established that the child had paralytic polio, felt alienated from a universe of "normal" experience and tended to see themselves as having been singled out for misfortune. We also pointed out that the families of the more seriously handicapped children tended to resort to such formulas as "There are others who are worse off" in attempting to find a symbolic resting place for themselves within some calculable scheme of human advantages and infirmities.

There remain, of course, the central questions of the handicapped status as such and the problems in self- and family identity to which it gives rise. How does the child see himself now that he is handicapped? How do his parents and others see him, and how do they interpret what they see? Can different patterns of perception and interpretation be delineated? If so, what are their significance, function, and practical implications? Although we have previously touched on several of these issues, we shall now deal with them more explicitly. Our discussion will be confined mainly to the nine families in which the child remained handicapped to some significant extent, for it is chiefly in these families that the issues with which we are here concerned had great meaning.

SOME REMARKS ON THE PROBLEM OF IDENTITY FOR THE HANDICAPPED

In considering the problems of identity confronting the handicapped person, one must view his situation alternately from the cultural and the individual standpoint. Unless he has been impaired from birth or early childhood, so that his primary identity is that of a handicapped person, it is more than likely that he will share, initially at least, many of the prejudiced and squeamish attitudes that are commonly shown toward the handicapped. He will tend, openly or secretly, to place a high value on many activities and pursuits that are closed to him because of his impairment. His attempts, if any, to be accepted by "normals" as "normal," are doomed to failure and frustration: not only do most "normals" find it difficult to include the handicapped person fully in their own category of being, but he himself, in that he shares the "normal" standards of personal evaluation, will in a sense support their rejection of him.[1] For the fact remains that, try as he may to hide or overlook it, he is at a distinct disadvantage with respect to several important values emphasized in our society: e.g., physical attractiveness; wholeness and symmetry of body parts; athletic prowess; and various physiognomic attributes felt to be prerequisite for a pleasant and engaging personality. The nine handicapped children in the study, for example, had to contend not only with visible distortions in body movement but also with braces, crutches, and other supportive appliances, appendages which many in the world of the unafflicted find disconcerting, "unnatural," and repugnant. The uneasiness that many "normals" feel in the company of a handicapped

[1] The social-psychological situation of the physically handicapped has been most thoroughly studied and written about by several students of the late Kurt Lewin, among them Roger G. Barker, Tamara Dembo, Lee Myerson, Ralph K. White, and Beatrice A. Wright. An excellent summary and reference source for the works of this group is Beatrice A. Wright, *Physical Disability—A Psychological Approach,* New York: Harper, 1960.

person is bound to affect his self-concept and to complicate in many ways his feelings of relatedness to "normals" in general.[2]

Interactionally, three alternative courses, or stratagems,[3] are open to the person faced with such a problem. Accepting "normal" standards and wishing to be viewed in terms of them, he and those intimately associated with him can attempt to eradicate or disguise the visible signs of the impairment so that others will not know that he is handicapped. In line with the analysis of similar phenomena in the field of race and ethnic relations, this stratagem might be termed "passing." Because of the gross apparency of their impairment, however, this alternative was closed to the nine handicapped children in the study, except for an occasional casual contact with a stranger or through a peculiar juxtaposition of circumstances. The purely fortuitous and fugitive opportunities available to the crippled person for the exercise of this stratagem are interestingly illustrated by the following incident, involving Marvin Harris. As a result of his refusal to wear his brace, Marvin broke his impaired leg in a fall, and the leg was placed temporarily in a long plaster cast. Marvin was not altogether unhappy about this, because when he was wearing the cast strangers often did not know that he was crippled. When Marvin was riding in a cab one day with his mother, the cab driver noticed the cast and asked, "How'd you break your leg, son? Playing football?" Mrs. Harris replied that this was indeed what had happened. When they got out of the cab Marvin said to his mother, "Am I glad you didn't tell him I had polio! They just think I have a broken leg."

Another stratagem open to the handicapped person and those close to him also entails no fundamental relinquishing of the normal standard. Without his attempting to pass, those aspects of his person that

---

[2] See Fred Davis, "Deviance Disavowal: The Management of Strained Interaction by the Visibly Handicapped," *Social Problems*, IX, 2 (Fall, 1961), 120-32.

[3] I choose the term "stratagem" in preference to type (or mode) of adjustment because it is less suggestive of a relative fixity or immutability in the interactional adaptation of the handicapped person. Especially in the beginning, the efforts of the nine children and their families to find ways of psychologically accommodating the physical deviance usually involved alternate testing and discarding of different adaptations, one frequently following on the heels of another. In view of this, it would be overstating the case to refer to these transistory adaptations as adjustments.

distinguish him from and cause him to be viewed as different by "normals" are made light of, rationalized in a variety of ways, viewed from a less disadvantageous perspective, and denied to be of any importance. This stratagem might be called "normalization."[4] Those who utilize this alternative seek to announce to others: "Though I may appear to be different, I really am not. Not only do I think of myself as normal, but others think of me as normal too." Seven-year-old Polly Manning, for example, decided to enter a contest sponsored by a magazine issued for handicapped children by a local welfare society. The contest asked the children to submit a name for the magazine. When Polly told her mother her first choice—"The Crippled Children's Book"—Mrs. Manning replied, "Well, that's right long. They said they wanted a short happy name, and that doesn't sound too happy." Polly then suggested "Cheer." With her mother's approval, this was the name she submitted.

The third interactional stratagem open to the handicapped person and those close to him might be called "disassociation." Unlike passing and normalization, disassociation generally involves some significant relinquishing of the normal standard, at least with respect to actual interaction, if not always at the level of personal ideology. Thus, while Marvin Harris never tired of proclaiming that he was "not really handicapped" and that he was "normal, like everyone else," all his actions—his avoidance of "normal" playmates and associations, his horror at having it become known that he wore a brace, etc.—belied these assertions. Families that disassociate typically seek to insulate themselves from events and involvements that might force them to recognize that others, and they themselves, regard the crippled child as "different."

Disassociation may take other forms, however, some of which could probably be regarded as more or less "healthy," depending on the standard of social adjustment invoked in the judgment. Among them are: (1) resentment and anger toward "normals" accompanied by feelings of self-hatred deriving from the person's inability to live up

[4] See F. Davis, "Deviance Disavowal," *op. cit.*, pp. 125-31, for an extended discussion of the concept of normalization. The concept was earlier used in a slightly different sense by Charlotte G. Schwartz, "Perspectives on Deviance—Wives' Definitions of Their Husbands' Mental Illness," *Psychiatry*, XX, 3 (August, 1957), 277-78.

to the prized normal standard;[5] (2) passive acceptance by the person of his exclusion from the world of "normals" punctuated periodically by attempts to ingratiate himself or to prove himself a "super nice guy"; (3) retreat to a more or less privatized sphere of hopes and fantasies in which the harsh impress of the normal standard is tenuously kept at bay; (4) an attempt to recast and reformulate personal values, activities, and associations so as to avoid or remove the sting from the often negative, condescending, and depreciating attitudes of "normals." The adoption of one of these forms of disassociation would not appear to preclude the adoption of another form at a later time or under altered circumstances. But, regardless of the particular form disassociation takes, what distinguishes it from the other stratagems is that, at the level of action, the person—much as he may prize or disdain the normal standard—does not base his behavior on the assumption that he will be responded to "normally" by "normals."

BECOMING A HANDICAPPED PERSON

The foregoing discussion may have suggested erroneously that the crippled person is faced with a fairly circumscribed choice among the three stratagems and that the choice is made mainly on the basis of tendencies existing in his personality. Although this may to some extent be true of an adolescent or adult who becomes handicapped— and who, it can be assumed, has had sufficient experience to enable him to inwardly rehearse the attitudes he will adopt—it is less clearly the case with children. What was striking about the group of nine handicapped children, particularly the youngest, was how long it took them to become aware of either the physical or the social implications of their situation. The following incident, by no means atypical, illustrates this point:

> Barely two months out of the hospital and wearing braces on both legs, seven-year-old Edward Short approached the coach of the local Little

[5] On the significance of the "normal standard" in handicapped-normal relations, see G. Ladieu, D. L. Adler, and T. Dembo, "Studies in Adjustment to Visible Injuries: Social Acceptance of the Injured," *Journal of Social Issues*, IV, 4 (1948), 55-61.

League baseball team and asked whether he could be put on the team. The coach, somewhat taken aback, handled the situation as best as he knew how and told Edward that all the positions on the team were filled for that year, advising him to inquire again the following year. Edward then went home and joyfully announced to his mother, much to her dismay, "I'll be playing with the Little Leaguers next year."

The unawareness of the children was no doubt influenced by other factors in addition to their lack of worldly experience. Some of these have been mentioned: the unqualified progress ideology of physiotherapy; the reluctance of doctors to give parents an unambiguous prognosis of the child's handicap; the parents' reluctance in turn to introduce the child to the social meanings of his handicap; and, finally, the tendency of many persons with whom the handicapped child comes in contact to, on the one hand, pretend not to notice his impairment while, on the other hand, acting in such a way as to show that they do.

The stratagem that child and family come to adopt for handling the problem of their relation to others involves more than the bringing to the surface of certain mechanisms latent in their personalities. In a deeper sense, the choice of stratagem, conscious or unwitting, emerges from their ongoing stream of social experience as they come to confront a new problem, the product being an attitudinal synthesis that derives from the impress of the responses of others on their historical self-concepts. Personality traits doubtless comprise a significant element in this developmental process, but to hold that they cause or explain the stratagem employed is a gross oversimplification.[6]

In the pages that follow we shall describe some of the initial experiences of the nine children in becoming identified as handicapped persons, grouping them under three headings: appearance, participation, and associations. Each, it will be noted, constitutes a communicative aspect of the self—i.e., a social medium, as it were, through which the child conveys "messages" about himself to others. Later we shall consider the stratagems that the children and their families employed in response.

[6] For one of the most prominent of the many studies based on this genre of analysis, see C. Landis and M. M. Bolles, *Personality and Sexuality in the Physically Handicapped Woman*, New York: Paul B. Hober, 1942.

Appearance

Physical appearance is perhaps the first realm in which the handicapped child begins to take significant notice of how he differs from other children. For all nine children, particularly the girls, the *literal* "looking-glass self"[7] that confronted them following their return from the hospital was one that they found difficult to accept as a true likeness of who and what they were. It was not uncommon for the child in these circumstances to fix on a particular piece of clothing in the hope that, if this could be made to approximate what other children wore, more essential aspects of the self would be transformed as well. For the girls, shoes typically became this object; much concern was expressed over when the orthopedic shoes could be discarded for low white or saddle shoes.

> As she was being dressed in her Easter finery by her mother, nine-year-old Norma Jean Mason gazed down at the bulge across her waist caused by the pelvic band. "Oh, this darn brace," she said. She then looked down at her feet, shod in plain, brown, high shoes of orthopedic construction to which the brace was attached. "If I could only have low white shoes with a buckle," she told her mother. Remarking on this incident, Mrs. Mason said, "She's always been particular about her clothes, but she didn't say too much about it. But I know she would have liked to have on what she's always been wearing."

Over a period of time, the sense of being different in appearance from other children received considerable validation for most of these children through their growing awareness of being stared at in a pitying, quizzical, or curious manner. Whenever Johnny Lawson sat down following class recitation he had to unhinge the knee lock on his brace. This made a clicking sound that caused all the boys who sat near him to look toward him and wait expectantly for the click. Being stared at and noticed became an extremely sensitive issue with the children, all the more so since there was very little they or their parents

[7] The conventional sociological use of the term refers to the image of self one acquires from others' reactions to one. (C. H. Cooley, *Human Nature and the Social Order*, New York: Scribner's, 1922.) See in this connection the interesting study of facial deformities by F. C. Macgregor, "Some Psycho-Social Problems Associated with Facial Deformities," *American Sociological Review*, XVI (October, 1951), 633.

could do to prevent it. The reaction of seven-year-old Laura Paulus to the following incident is symbolic of the growing dilemma of marginal identification they experienced. Riding in the family automobile one afternoon, the Pauluses passed a woman who wore a brace walking on the road. Laura exclaimed, "See that lady! I didn't stare at that lady!"

Participation

In other connections we have pointed to the many serious problems of participation confronting the nine handicapped children. These included a wide range of juvenile activities, such as ball playing, roller skating, bike riding, dancing, and swimming. For many of them it extended to numerous nonrecreational spheres as well—e.g., attending a regular school, using public transportation, ascending and descending stairs. To participate is literally "to be a part of," and for several children the inability to play their part in full accordance with the normal standard led them increasingly to disassociate themselves from such activities. Marvin Harris, for example, would spend long hours at home "playing ball" by himself. He would bounce the ball off the walls and furniture, frequently smashing dishes, picture frames, light fixtures, and bric-a-brac. When asked by his parents to take the ball outside, Marvin would refuse angrily and grow even more destructive in his play. His vehemence suggested that he did not regard himself as fit to be seen in public participating in so "normal" a boyish pursuit as playing ball.

The majority of the children did participate to some extent in play and games with non-handicapped children following their discharge from the hospital. Almost without exception, however, such participation was, as indicated, of an adaptive variety. Participation of this type naturally had the effect of placing the handicapped child in a decidedly marginal position with respect to his playmates. After a time it was not uncommon for them to include or exclude him as whim and opportunity moved them. As Mr. Lawson described his son's play with neighborhood children:

> Sometimes they'll just say they don't have room for anyone, and they'll say, "Well, you can't play." They'll play baseball in the alley where it requires hitting and running, and they have the same amount on each

team and sometimes they'll say, "Well, you can be catcher for both teams." It's more or less a mood they get in, don't you think? Lots of times something will happen like that and he'll sit here and watch them or, in other words, be on the sidelines.

Because the families were followed for only a short time after the child returned home, it would be impossible for us to assess the long-range consequences of this kind of marginal participation for the self-concept of the child. It cannot be doubted, however, that it raises serious obstacles to satisfactory identification with "normal" children.

Associations

An inseparable part of the identity problem posed for the handicapped child is the question of his peer associations: who his friends are, the kind of relationship he has with them, and how this is altered as a result of his being perceived as handicapped.[8] Although our data on these questions are not wholly comparable,[9] they strongly suggest that the friendship patterns of the handicapped children were greatly affected by their experience. Unmistakable evidence of this was found in the records of four of the nine children who remained significantly handicapped during the post-hospital period.[10] It is illustrated most strikingly in the case of Norma Jean Mason, a ten-year-old who returned from the hospital to the same stable, working- and lower-middle-class neighborhood in which she had lived since birth.

[8] For an interesting account of the segregated friendship patterns that obtain among handicapped and non-handicapped children "integrated" in the same elementary-school classes, see D. G. Force, "Social Status of Physically Handicapped Children," *Exceptional Children*, XXIII (December, 1956), 104-07.

[9] For example, three of the children moved to new neighborhoods at some point following their return from the hospital. Although the ensuing friendship patterns of these children also appeared qualitatively different from what they had been prior to the illness, it is difficult to know how much of the change can be attributed to the handicap and how much to the readjustments inevitably occasioned by a change of neighborhood.

[10] Of the remaining five, three appear to have been too young (five and six years of age) to have developed a stable circle of friends prior to their illness. A fourth child lived both prior and subsequent to his hospitalization in neighborhoods of high residential turnover. The family of the fifth withdrew from the study before useful data could be obtained.

Of the several neighborhood friends with whom Norma Jean played before her illness, Sally and Eleanor were by far the closest. All during the time Norma Jean was in the hospital, these two were extremely attentive and solicitous, writing her frequently, sending gifts, and inquiring almost daily of Mrs. Mason how Norma Jean was progressing. On the weekend visits home that Norma Jean made prior to her discharge, Sally and Eleanor spent almost all their free time with her and often accompanied her back to the hospital in the Mason family car.

Less than two months after her discharge, changes were already evident in Norma Jean's relationship with these and other neighborhood children. According to Mrs. Mason, Eleanor had more or less completely "drifted away," while Sally came to play with Norma Jean much less frequently than she had previously. This hurt Norma Jean, and she would often ask Mrs. Mason why Sally did not visit when she expected her to. Wishing to protect Norma Jean's feelings, Mrs. Mason would tell her, "Well, maybe her mother has something for her to do. She has a small brother and she might have to mind him. Why don't you call her up to see if she can come over?" When Norma Jean would call, as often as not Sally would have some excuse for not being able to come—homework, an errand to run for her mother, babysitting with her little brother. Sally never reciprocated by calling Norma Jean and inviting her to her house. At about this time, Norma Jean began to play dodgeball in front of the Mason home with several of the younger children in the neighborhood, who were apparently flattered by the unaccustomed attentions of an older child.

In the months that followed, Norma Jean saw less and less of Sally and instead became very friendly with a somewhat older (12 years) neighborhood girl named Gloria. Norma Jean had known Gloria before her illness but she, Eleanor, and Sally did not especially like Gloria and frequently excluded her from their favorite activities. Now Norma Jean and Gloria were fast friends, Gloria accompanying her almost everywhere, helping her with her wheelchair, and doing whatever she could to make things easier for Norma Jean. As Mrs. Mason described the relationship, "She's like a mother to Norma Jean." According to Mrs. Mason, Norma Jean knew this and took advantage of it by having Gloria do many things for her that she could easily do for herself.

The close friendship between the two girls lasted through the summer, but with the arrival of fall Gloria's visits became much less frequent. Mrs. Mason attributed this to Gloria's growing interest in boys and her corresponding loss of interest in female companionship. On occasion

Gloria still would swoop down on Norma Jean, suddenly and unannounced, and try to inject their relationship with some of its former enthusiasm. After several such attempts Gloria ceased trying to make amends and thereafter the two girls saw each other only rarely.

Throughout this period, however, Norma Jean slowly—and, at first, very cautiously—began making friends at the school for handicapped children she attended. During her first semester there she joined the glee club and began having regular twice-a-week phone chats with one of her classmates. For some time, though, neither visited the other's house. In the fall of that year Norma Jean began inviting this girl and several others from her class to her home for weekend parties, garden picnics, and record-listening sessions.

The last time the family was seen, some sixteen months after Norma Jean's discharge, a somewhat mixed pattern obtained with respect to her friendship pattern. During the school week she still on occasion played dodgeball or some other game with several of the neighborhood children, but in a much more casual and disinterested way than before. Her important recreations were more and more reserved for weekends, when she would gather with her girl friends from the school for handicapped children. Moreover, her two friendship circles remained strictly segregated; apart from herself, no child who belonged to one also belonged to the other. This did not mean, however, that Norma Jean had lost interest in her neighborhood friends. Increasingly, though, when she made overtures in their direction, she discovered that they were going off on activities in which she could not participate. As Mrs. Mason reported, "She still sees the girls going off, or she'll call them up and ask if they're going to the show today, or what are they going to do, and they'll say, 'Well, we're going ice skating.' Well, I imagine she's bound to feel hurt inside in some way."

Judging from Norma Jean's experience and that of the other children who returned as "altered persons" to their old friends and pastimes, it would appear that there is no sudden and sharp break with former peers and no quickly consummated induction into a new subculture of handicapped persons. Instead, what happened might be described as a gradual, socially coerced process of downward mobility in the "normal" peer group, one that repeatedly posed for the child the same questions of identity and belongingness. For these children, the discovery of a new set of associates and new definitions of the self was intermittent, tentative, and at first highly experimental in character.[11]

Most striking in this connection was the tendency of the child, following his initial exclusion from the center of the peer group's activities, to form a close friendship with another child whose status and acceptance in the group was also marginal. Thus we observe Norma Jean Mason's developing relationship with the formerly excluded Gloria. Similarly, when his neighborhood friends would no longer play baseball with him, Eddie Short became quite intimate with a boy whom Eddie's parents described as "a little childish, and not at all interested in sports like Eddie." Johnny Lawson's mother reported that Johnny gradually gave up the "wild bunch of boys" he used to play with and formed a friendship with a more placid and studious lad. Whether such marginal friendships function as a temporary way station in a life-career passage to a new, handicap-oriented identity or endure as a kind of socially marginal sequestering place, neither wholly within nor wholly without the world of "normal" peers, is a fascinating and important question. Unfortunately, the children could not be followed for a long enough time to provide us with answers to it.

NORMALIZATION AND DISASSOCIATION

The strains on identity experienced by child and family in the spheres of appearance, participation, and associations were psychologically counterbalanced to varying degrees by the employment of interactional stratagems of the types discussed earlier. Of the stratagems available to the families, normalization was resorted to more extensively, as Table 2 (page 159) shows. Whether its primary stratagem was normalization or disassociation, however, instances of the use of both stratagems could be found in each family. In the following case histories, that of the Pauluses shows how normalization was utilized to a

---

[11] Although in response to very different kinds of pressures, this "becoming" process of affiliation and identification is similar in its general outlines to that depicted for recruitment into a wide variety of deviant subcultures. See, for example, A. Lindesmith, *Opiate Addiction,* Bloomington, Ind.: Principia Press, 1947, and H. S. Becker, "Becoming a Marihuana User," *American Journal of Sociology,* LIX (November, 1953), 235-42.

striking degree. In the second, that of the Harrises, disassociation was favored.

The Pauluses—A Case of Pronounced Normalization

Six-year-old Laura Paulus was without doubt the most handicapped child in the group of nine. She wore full-length braces on both legs, a pelvic band, high orthopedic shoes, and, when traveling more than a short distance, had to use crutches as well. Neither the doctors nor the physiotherapist who treated her at the hospital held out a favorable prognosis, although they did indicate that certain minor improvements in functional capacity might result from later corrective surgery. Needless to say, from a purely physical standpoint Laura was extremely limited in what she could do. Her movements were slow and awkward, and such games as she could engage in with other children required considerable adaptation and amendment.

In view of Laura's condition, it might be supposed that her situation was rife for disassociative tendencies; that, because of her grave inability to keep up with other children, she would soon be excluded, or would voluntarily withdraw, from the group of neighborhood children with whom she had played prior to her illness. But during the two years in which the Pauluses were seen, nothing of the kind happened, thanks chiefly to the efforts and personality of Mrs. Paulus, a young and energetic woman whom Laura admired immensely and whose guidance Laura seemed ever-ready to follow with equanimity and good cheer.

No sooner was Laura out of the hospital than Mrs. Paulus re-registered her in the school she had attended before her illness. Unlike most of the other parents in the study, she did this without first consulting the hospital doctors on the possibility or appropriateness of doing so. (Parents of children less severely handicapped than Laura were advised to enroll their child in a school for handicapped children.) Despite the girl's condition, Mrs. Paulus also saw to it that no unusual arrangements were made to get Laura to and from school, because, as she stated, she wanted Laura to follow as normal a school routine as possible. Laura therefore used regular city bus service. However, she was accompanied by, and quite dependent on, a classmate friend who held her books for her, helped her up and down the boarding platform, paid her fare, and guided her to a seat.

Mrs. Paulus also saw to it that Laura's play and social life were kept "as normal as possible." The first weeks following Laura's return from the hospital were filled with children's parties and other festivities in the Paulus home in honor of Laura's homecoming. Mrs. Paulus always encouraged Laura to go out and play with the neighborhood children, even though she knew that it was difficult for Laura to keep up and that it was necessary for them to adapt games in order to accommodate her. In this connection, Mrs. Paulus remarked, with considerable pride, "She really mixes with the other children. They seem to include her in everything they do." Later that year she enrolled Laura in the local Brownie troop, and although Laura could not, for example, go on hikes, on such occasions Mrs. Paulus would drive her to the camp site after the other children had arrived there on foot.

Several somewhat atypical circumstances, it should be noted, helped Mrs. Paulus initially to normalize her daughter's situation to such a pronounced extent. The Pauluses lived in an unusually close-knit and community-spirited neighborhood of detached working- and lower-middle-class homes. Laura was well known and liked, and the neighbors along with their children seemed more than ordinarily inclined to go out of their way to accommodate her. Also, Mrs. Paulus was active in a number of church and service organizations in the community. This brought the family's situation to the sympathetic attention of numerous local persons and groups. The Pauluses, therefore, were not forgotten so soon after their child's homecoming as were other families in the study.

At least in her contacts with the project staff, Mrs. Paulus always exuded an air of optimism. Laura, she maintained, was "doing beautifully" and led "as normal and happy a life as any other child." She cited as "proof" the many "normal" activities Laura engaged in. Mr. Paulus, although privately neither so optimistic nor so enthusiastic as his wife—once, for example, he spoke of his great disillusionment when he lifted one of Laura's legs and "it felt like a piece of rubber hanging there"—was careful not to express his misgivings before Laura or his wife.

Despite Mrs. Paulus' often strenuous efforts to normalize her daughter's situation, there were of course times when Laura could or would not be treated as a "normal" girl, and when the pretense of such treatment came dangerously near breaking down or actually did so. Several incidents point up the "fatal flaw" of normalization as a deviance-correcting stratagem: the fact that others are frequently unable or unwilling to go along with it. Thus, for example, at an Elks-sponsored "kiddie show" at the local movie house, Laura was conspicuously given many more gifts than the other children. She was not permitted to take her seat until all the other children were seated, and after the film was over the children were made to remain in their seats until Laura departed. Again, when the Pauluses made a sightseeing trip to Washington, D.C., Laura insisted on negotiating the long flight of steps leading up to the Capitol without her parents' assistance. After watching her laborious ascent for several minutes, a bystander turned scoldingly on Mr. and Mrs. Paulus and said, "Are you going to make that poor child walk up all those steps by herself?"

Mrs. Paulus' plan to have Laura travel to school "normally" came to an end one day when the school principal saw Laura struggling to alight from a bus. Over Mrs. Paulus' protests, he insisted that he could not assume responsibility for Laura's welfare on or near the school grounds if she continued to use public transportation. Either Laura would have to travel by specially arranged taxicab service (for which the school would pay) or she would have to be sent to a school for handicapped children. Faced with this choice, Mrs. Paulus reluctantly consented to have a cab call for Laura every morning and bring her home every afternoon.

As a rule, however, Mrs. Paulus rationalized or made light of those occasions when the normalization formula broke down. For example, after the "kiddie show" at which Laura had been singled out for special treatment by the Elks representative, Mrs. Paulus remarked laughingly, "Everywhere Laura goes, all the men are after her." When Laura, against the advice of doctor and physiotherapist, began to gain too much weight, thereby putting an added strain on her impaired extremities, Mrs. Paulus spoke of her intention of putting Laura on a diet, because, she said, she did not want to see her "lose her cute little figure."

Serving as a character model for Mrs. Paulus throughout much of this period was an ex-polio case whom she had met through her church circle. Mrs. Paulus said of this woman:

> People I have come in contact with always say that she forgets about polio. She completely forgets that she even has braces. She minds her own business. She went to high school and college. She took a lot of chemistry and she has one daughter, twelve years old, I believe. She told me, "I owe all that to my family for pushing me and making me go right along doing whatever my sister did. They didn't treat me any different than they did my sister. She went to dances and different things at school. If she went, my parents made me go too." . . . I sort of feel that way, too. I just feel like, well I'll let Laura go that way, because it's going to mean an awful lot to her.

The Harrises—A Case of Disassociation

Although eleven-year-old Marvin Harris was not so severely handicapped as several other children in the group (his right lower extremity was affected, and he wore a full-length brace and pelvic band), he and his family appeared to react more profoundly and with greater distress to Marvin's polio and subsequent impairment than did any other family in the study. This was evident from the very first interview, when Mrs. Harris wept and kept repeating, "I don't want my son to be a cripple." Mr. Harris wallowed in self-punitive memories of a polio-crippled acquaintance of his youth who, he said, was mean, embittered, and disliked by all who knew him. Marvin, too, at the beginning of his hospitalization, evidenced near-panic at the thought of braces and crippling, and on more than one occasion his mother had to reassure him that his affected leg would not grow thinner than the other.

During the course of hospitalization, however, Marvin calmed down considerably. After some difficulty with a couple of other boys on the ward, he was moved to a private room where he spent most of the day watching television and visiting for brief periods with other children. When he received his brace and crutches prior to discharge he did not seem particularly upset, which perhaps accounts for the very favorable report that treatment personnel gave of him at about this time. They described Marvin as a serious, intelligent lad who was well motivated and had a good understanding of his condition and of the limitations it imposed. They viewed his apparently mature reaction to bracing as a good augury of his post-hospital adjustment.

A more inaccurate prediction could hardly have been made. In a host of ways, Marvin and his parents soon made it apparent that his handicap was fundamentally unacceptable to them, despite the parents' assertion that they would do everything possible to make Marvin happy.

On the doctor's recommendation, Mrs. Harris enrolled Marvin, very much against his wishes, in a school for handicapped children. Marvin not only resisted attending this school but, when it became apparent that he had no other choice, pleaded unsuccessfully with his father to drive him there every day so that he would not be seen in company with other handicapped children on the school bus. During the year he attended this school, Marvin formed no friendships there and did everything possible to isolate himself from his handicapped classmates. He vehemently rejected the offer of a social worker to send him, at her agency's expense, to a summer camp for handicapped children for an eight-week vacation. Except for one occasion when, in a rage, he reportedly shouted, "I'm not like other children" in response to his mother's plea that he "behave nice like other children," Marvin constantly protested that he was "not really handicapped" and saw no reason for attending a school for handicapped children.

In view of their repeated protestations that he was "not like those other handicapped children," it might be assumed that Marvin and his parents would do everything possible to normalize his situation and to deny or minimize the social and interactional significance of his impairment. The contrary proved to be the case. Marvin's keen sense of stigma and resultant self-hatred led him—often with the tacit support of his parents—to reject "normals" as well as other handicapped children. The following incidents are revealing in this connection.

A few weeks after Marvin returned from the hospital, his family moved to a new neighborhood which, although it contained several elementary schools and a high school, was described by Mrs. Harris as a "middle-aged neighborhood," with no other boys with whom Marvin could play. In the same interview, however, Mrs. Harris reported that Marvin had turned away and pretended to tie his shoe when he saw two boys his own age approaching from the other end of the street. In subsequent interviews it came out that Marvin had been approached several times by a neighborhood boy with a speech defect who wanted Marvin to join the local Boy Scout troop (non-handicapped) to which he belonged. Perhaps resenting the overtures of a somewhat less than "normal" emissary, Marvin rejected the boy's invitations and made it plain that he wished to have nothing to do with him or his friends. Another time Marvin made a half-hearted attempt to resume friendship with a boy from his old neighborhood. Despite the fact that on several occasions the boy traveled a considerable distance to accompany Marvin to the movies, Marvin soon stopped seeing him. He claimed that the boy "only wanted someone to go to the movies with" and was not "a real friend."

It is interesting to note that the disassociation fostered by Marvin in his own relationships was experienced by the parents in theirs as well. During Marvin's hospital stay and subsequently, Mrs. Harris' brothers and sisters and their families telephoned, visited, and invited the Harrises less and less frequently. As Mrs. Harris put it, "I think that people think when they go to see somebody like that they're going to see somebody that's abnormal or something, and they're afraid to look." Mrs. Harris' mother had often advised her children that she wanted "only good things to hear, the bad things don't tell me." Apparently Marvin's situation was thought to fit the latter category.

The interviewer noted that Marvin did not so much deny his impairment as reject it. Several months out of the hospital, in defiance of the warnings of the doctors, he took to discarding his brace at the slightest opportunity. He would hide it under a pile of clothes in the closet when he knew company was coming; he would leave it lying about wherever he happened to drop it after coming into the house; he was even averse to having Mrs. Harris' brother and his four-year-old cousin, both of whom lived with the Harrises, see him wearing it. In restaurants and other public places Marvin would sit so that his body shielded his braced leg from the view of others. During the summer months, the Harrises made many trips to the beach. Marvin would refuse adamantly to go along if his parents made him wear the brace. Invariably, they gave in to the demand, and it was on one such occasion that Marvin broke his impaired leg, when a child running past caused him to lose his balance and fall. Following this incident—

the parents and Marvin were severely reprimanded by the doctors because he had not worn his brace—it seemed for a time that Marvin's attitude had changed. (He was so penitent and guilty that for several days after the accident Mr. and Mrs. Harris worried over whether he would ever have the courage to lift himself out of the sick bed again.) A few months later, however, he was again refusing successfully to wear his brace.

Throughout this period Mr. and Mrs. Harris complained to the interviewer of the difficulty of controlling Marvin and getting him to do "what's best for him." At the same time, they appeared tacitly to support and encourage much of the behavior of which they complained. They were immensely indulgent of Marvin. For example, they were constantly giving him extra money so that he could buy sweets and other between-meal snacks. On the rare occasions when the parents went out for the evening, they left large quantities of delicatessen for Marvin in case he became hungry, depressed, or restless. With his parents away Marvin's spirits always did flag, and when they returned he would scold them for not having left more food. (Quite stout before polio, Marvin grew excessively fat as a result of these indulgences. Although the doctors constantly warned Mrs. Harris to put Marvin on a diet, she apparently took the view that this would exact much too high a psychic price from her and from Marvin.) In time, Marvin grew increasingly indignant whenever his parents decided to go out for the evening. Once, after they left despite his threats, he rushed to his room in a fury and addressed a letter to them in which he wrote, "I wish both of you would die in two minutes." Mrs. Harris later expressed bewilderment to the interviewer over why Marvin would do such a thing.

In more calm and considered moments Mr. and Mrs. Harris would assert, as did Marvin, that he "really wasn't handicapped." Mrs. Harris stated, "He's nothing like those cerebral-palsy kids and children without arms or legs that go to school with him." Resorting to a kind of second-order normalization formula, Mrs. Harris would try to explain away Marvin's extremely negative and rebellious behavior by claiming, "All boys his age are that way. My sister's boy gives her a lot of trouble too, so I guess it's only normal." Rationalizations of this kind were doubtless comforting to Mrs. Harris in view of her often-expressed suspicion that the gods had visited a terrible misfortune upon her, one that she had to suffer in silence because of the weakness and ineptitude of the other members of the family. At one point she stated:

> My husband is, I think, affected more than anybody. He's just being eaten up inside because of Marvin, and although I feel very badly about it, I always have my hopes. But he just doesn't seem to. You can just see how badly he feels, and I think he is getting very, very nervous from it. He can't seem to take it at all. . . . Marvin falls once in a while and he has to pick him up, and after that he just doesn't seem to be—it seems to take an awful lot out of him, because he realizes how helpless Marvin is.

A year out of the hospital, Marvin still had made no friends, either at school or in the neighborhood. Occasionally he visited one of his cousins, but this was more a matter of family connivance than spontaneous friendship. Otherwise, the only other children he played with were his six-year-old brother, Keith, and some of Keith's friends. More and more, Marvin took to accompanying his mother on her late-afternoon visits to women friends. Although he often sulked, behaved offensively, and claimed not to enjoy these visits, he was even more bitter when Mrs. Harris did not offer to take him. At home Marvin, as has been noted, often acted with a kind of determined destructiveness, bouncing a ball off the walls of the apartment and "accidentally" smashing vases, lamps, picture frames, and bric-a-brac. The only compensatory interest that he evidenced was a sporadic involvement in modeling sailing vessels and airplanes. Most of his non-school time was spent in watching television. Mrs. Harris once remarked that television had been the most important factor in helping Marvin, both in the hospital and, later, at home.

Although Marvin's physical condition had shown scarcely any improvement, when last seen Mr. and Mrs. Harris had found new hope in anticipating Marvin's imminent enrollment in a "regular" local high school. Marvin also was highly pleased with this development. His parents took the view that Marvin was at last receiving his due, since they—but more especially, he—were still inclined to maintain that he was "not really handicapped like the others." In apparent disregard of all that had happened during the year, Mrs. Harris remarked enthusiastically, "I think that when he goes to a regular school, he'll feel that he's just like everybody else."

The Harrises and Pauluses represent extremes in the range of adjustment stratagems found among the nine families whose children remained significantly handicapped. None of the others disassociated or normalized to so pronounced a degree, and even these two families on occasion displayed behavior befitting the other stratagem. Viewing the group as a whole, we find a graduated distribution of mixed stratagems, with some families resorting to normalization more than disassociation, and others vice versa. This combination of apparently opposing psychological tendencies is, we venture, characteristic of a great number of adjustment processes, particularly those emanating from new and unfamiliar situations such as those we are dealing with here.

What, then, can we say about the actual distribution of adaptive stratagems among the nine families? What factors account for or are significantly implicated in the relative partiality accorded normalization as against disassociation, and vice versa? Table 2 addresses itself to these questions, although it must be remembered that, because of the small numbers involved, the findings are at best suggestive rather than conclusive.

We note first that normalization was the favored stratagem. Six of the families are ranged along this end of the continuum, whereas only three tend toward disassociation. Other things being equal, this is perhaps to be expected in view of our society's pronounced idealization of the normal, the healthy, the physically attractive. As has been noted by such students of contemporary American culture as Riesman, Mead, and Gorer, as a people we are suspicious of most forms of eccentricity; we tend to recoil from manifestations that depart from a relatively narrow social definition of "the normal," be they of a moral, characterological, or physical bent. Hence, it can be hypothesized that, as representative bearers of this ethos, the families found it easier and morally more acceptable to assimilate the social deviance latent in the child's handicap to the cultural framework of "normal" aspirations and imagery already internalized by them. Normalization proved the favored scheme in that, without going so far as to deny the existence of the physical handicap, it sought to sustain the "democratic" fiction that the impairment was of no consequence in social relations and that the child was, for all practical purposes, "normal, like everyone else."

But, as can be inferred from Table 2, the difficulty with this kind of psycho-cultural explanation is that, while it may shed some light on the gross tendency toward normalization among the families as a whole, it does not account for the differences among them. Not all the families were normalizers, and even among the six who were, there were decided differences in degree. It is necessary, therefore, to seek additional factors that can better delineate the range of adjustments uncovered. Of the many situational and structural factors that suggest themselves in this connection and that could be put to the test, only four were found to be of potential significance: degree of handicap; age of child at time of discharge; sibling constellation; and style of family functioning.[12]

Regarding these we find in Table 2 a striking uniformity among the three families falling within the disassociation half of the continuum. In each the child was seriously handicapped; he was between 9 and 12 years of age; he was either an only child or was more than five years older or younger than his nearest sib; and last, his family was relatively traditional, as opposed to equalitarian, in its life style. For their part, the six families in the normalization half of the continuum reveal almost as much uniformity. With two exceptions, these were all children who were moderately handicapped. All six were young (between 5 and 8 years), and all had at least one sibling no more than five years older or younger. All but two came from equalitarian family settings. Although the data permit us to offer only plausible, rather than definitive, explanations of these findings, it is worth while

[12] Other factors that were tested for and found insignificant were: sex of child; number of children in family; religion; residential stability; economic stability and type of neighborhood lived in (apartment area, single- and two-family homes, relatively open country). This does not, of course, preclude the possibility that certain of these factors, or still others, would emerge as significant were a larger number of families studied. In addition, certain obvious factors (e.g., socioeconomic level, parental education, ethnicity) could not be tested for meaningfully because the families differed so little in these respects.

TABLE 2

Normalization-Disassociation Tendencies in the Nine Families

Favored Stratagem[a]	STRUCTURAL AND SITUATIONAL ATTRIBUTES							
	Moderately handicapped	Aged 5-8 at discharge	One or more sibs within 5 yrs. in age	Equalitarian family life style[b]	Seriously handicapped	Aged 9-12 at discharge	No sibs within 5 yrs. in age	Traditional family life style[c]
Normalization (Pronounced)								
Paulus		X	X	X	X			
(Dominant)								
Lawson	X	X	X					X
Short	X	X	X					X
(Tendency)								
Johnson	X	X	X	X				
Prince	X	X	X	X				
Manning		X	X	X	X			
Disassociation (Tendency)								
Mason					X	X	X	X
Stewart					X	X	X	X
(Dominant)								
Harris					X	X	X	X

[a] Ranking of families is based on summary evaluations of a variety of behavioral and attitudinal responses to the child's handicap: e.g., extent and type of peer associations of child; child's participation in or withdrawal from a normal round of activities; degree and type of special treatment accorded child by parents; expressed attitudes toward the social meanings of the handicap; relative presence or absence of sense of stigma.

[b] Based on three factors: (1) wife's having worked since marriage; (2) a fairly loose sexual division of tasks and responsibilities in the family; and (3) no evidence of extensive parental involvement with kin, particularly with those in family of orientation. Where there was a 2-1 split among the criteria, the family was classified according to the two in which it led.

[c] The converse of [b].

to consider briefly how each of the factors may be related to the preference shown by a family for normalization or disassociation.

Concerning degree of handicap, it might be argued that the more
severely handicapped the child is, the fewer the opportunities offered
him and his family to normalize their situation. Whereas the moderately handicapped child can as a rule attend a regular school and
participate in neighborhood play to some extent, these normalizing
opportunities are usually closed to the seriously handicapped child.
The result is that, even where a predisposition to normalization exists,
the absence of tangible opportunities in the social environment induces
disassociative tendencies in the family.

Of the four factors, the age of the victim and its proximity to that
of his siblings, if any, are the two that most consistently differentiate
the choice of adaptive stratagem (Table 2). Regarding the age factor,
we can only repeat a familiar observation of rehabilitation workers to
the effect that it is generally not until the child approaches adolescence
that his impairment acquires a deep significance in the eyes of his
peers. Since normalization requires at least the appearance of acceptance by "normal" peers, it can be postulated that as the child nears
adolescence problems of physical attractiveness and sex begin to loom
large, and he or she is excluded increasingly by peers from a normal
round of activities.[13] Like the seriously handicapped child, the older
handicapped child is confronted with a reduced range of opportunities
for employing normalization techniques and hence is driven in a disassociative direction.

As for the relationship noted between sibling constellation and
choice of adaptive stratagem, we would hypothesize that this is due to
the difference in the situational and moral constraints generated in
multi-sibling families with children of approximately the same age as
compared with only-child families or families in which sibs are widely
spaced in age. As was suggested earlier, in multi-sib families, parents,
for both practical and moral reasons, are likely to espouse a policy of
equal treatment toward all the children, regardless of the somewhat
unique considerations pertaining to the handicapped child. Because it
is easier to treat the handicapped child as if he were "normal" than to
treat the others as if they were handicapped, as a corrective stratagem

[13] See the account of Norma Jean Mason's experience with neighborhood
peers, pp. 145-47.

normalization suits such families. Where there are no sibs or where a relatively large span of years separates the handicapped child from his nearest sib, parents are less likely to feel constraints of this type and thus are freer to treat the child in specially protective, indulgent, or other particularized ways. As is so strikingly shown in the Harris case, this special treatment usually serves to re-enforce whatever disassociation tendencies exist in the family.

Finally, there is the more complex matter of style of family functioning, although this is less consistently associated with choice of adaptive stratagem than are the other factors. To the degree that the equalitarian style is related to normalization, and the traditional to disassociation, we would reason as follows. Since normalization entails a certain flexibility in interpersonal relations[14]—i.e., the capacity to sustain "as if" reformulations of persons and events—the equalitarian family atmosphere, with its looser differentiation of family roles and greater tolerance of pluralistic demands, offers a more fertile medium for the cultivation of normalization techniques than does the traditional family atmosphere. By comparison, the latter, with its stricter demarcation of age-sex roles and harsher standards of acceptable performance, is less capable of accommodating the "slippage" from conventional normative standards that normalization entails. Feeling great shame and estrangement in its misfortune, the traditionally oriented family is likely to move out reactively in a disassociative direction.

Obviously, the foregoing hypotheses do not exhaust the many possible causes underlying the phenomenon represented in Table 2. (How, for example, are we to account for the fact that while the paired attributes seem clearly to distinguish the normalizers from the disassociators, in themselves they contribute so little to an understanding of the gradations found *within* each classification?) As is often the case with complex behavioral patterns of this type, it is doubtful whether any single set of independent factors can ever account fully for the distribution of cases along a dependent variable. There are always "other factors" which come into play but which escape detection or measurement. It is hoped, however, that the analysis presented here will at least sensitize future investigators to the social-structural

[14] Cf. Davis, "Deviance Disavowal," *op. cit.,* pp. 126-30.

and situational—in addition to the intrapsychic—sources of adaptation in the family.

CHANGE AND CONTINUANCE OF IDENTITY

A further comment is in order before closing this discussion of the identity problems of the families. Despite the obvious and sometimes abrupt changes in the family's scheme of life occasioned by the child's handicap, it was remarkable how little conscious or explicit awareness of such changes the families demonstrated. Each time a parent was interviewed, he was asked whether anything seemed changed, whether anyone in the family felt or acted differently toward the handicapped child, whether the child acted or felt differently about himself. Almost invariably, although sometimes only after a puzzled silence, the answers would come back that nothing was changed, that no one in the family felt or acted differently toward anyone else, and that the handicapped child was much the same child he had always been. Were it not for the parents' incidental remarks and unreflecting reports on specific events and situations, one might not have surmised that there had been any significant alteration in their lives. The disquieting apprehension of one's self-in-change that experiences of this magnitude are known to evoke in some persons was here muted by a sense of sameness and unbroken continuity with the past.

The social scientist cannot help but point to the many positive social functions served by so steadfast a continuity of identity.[15]

[15] With a few notable exceptions, social psychologists have neglected the manifold issues of continuity and change of identity. The two levels of the problem—the changes actually wrought in the person's life scheme and the quality of his comprehension and appreciation of them—have been badly blurred. It is implicitly assumed in many analyses either that (1) the objective changes are of little consequence if there is no subjective recognition of them or (2) the failure of recognition is irrational or pathological, and hence indicative only of an ego-defensive need to distort "reality." Rarely is it considered that the lag or disjunction between change and its conscious apprehension may serve important adaptive functions, both for the person and for his social group: viz., the maintenance of a necessary degree of continuity in self-conception and the preservation of sufficient expectational stability among those with whom the person customarily interacts. See Strauss, *op. cit.*, pp. 141-47; Erik H. Erikson, "Identity and the Life Cycle," *Psychological Issues* I, Monograph No. 1 (1959); Harold Garfinkel, "The Rational Properties of Scientific and Common Sense Activities," *Behavioral Science* V, 1 (January, 1960), 72-82.

Among other things, it helps to moor persons and groups psychologically in ways that inure them to the potentially too disruptive effects of change. The humanist, on the other hand, viewing this same phenomenon from the ethic of a higher sensibility, is bound to see it as a hindrance to self-understanding and hence as damaging to man's deepest creative impulses. Be this as it may, interviews with these families often suggested the inverse of a familiar aphorism: *plus c'est la même chose, plus ça change.*

SUMMARY

The fundamental issue of identity confronting the families of the handicapped children was how to view, interpret, and respond to the many negative meanings imputed to a visible physical handicap in our society. Two broad strategems of adjustment, normalization and disassociation, were found. Families that tended toward normalization denied the manifest social significance of the handicap rather than the handicap itself; they would explain it away, make light of it, and, most of all, attempt to validate socially the claim that others as well as they themselves viewed their child as "normal." Families that leaned toward disassociation sought to insulate themselves from contacts, situations, and involvements which might force them to recognize that others, and they themselves, regarded the crippled child as somehow "different." Both strategems, of course, had inherent limitations and from time to time broke down, sometimes resoundingly.

Although no family normalized or disassociated exclusively, some tended more to normalization, others more to disassociation. Although it is impossible to determine the precise combination of factors that might account for the relative degrees of normalization and disassociation evinced by the families, in general the following situational and structural attributes appear to be associated with the respective strategems: Normalization was found in families in which the polio child was relatively young, only moderately handicapped, and closely related in age to one or more siblings, and whose family functioned in a more or less equalitarian fashion. Disassociation was found when the polio child was older, severely handicapped, and either an only child or far removed in age from his nearest sibling, and whose family functioned in a more traditional fashion.

As regards their over-all interpretation of the quality and meaning of their situation, all the parents were wont to claim, despite much objective evidence to the contrary, that the experience had resulted in no significant changes in their lives or in the attitudes and behavior of family members toward one another. This strong sense of continuity of identity in the midst of change doubtless betokens a high degree of social stability in these families. But from another vantage point, it perhaps also testifies to a failure of creative impulse—an excessive contentment with the familiar and known that inhibits the discovery of new meanings and purposes when important life circumstances change.

I_N

Chapter 7. Implications

following the 14 families to this point in their history we have touched on many areas of sociological interest, each of which might have been subjected to analysis in its own right were it not for the naturalistic method that has guided this narration. This method has both advantages and disadvantages. On the one hand, it helps to check the tendency to so reify abstract and classificatory indices of the phenomena studied that they come to serve as substitutes for concrete explanations of the phenomena themselves. On the other hand, the attempt to present a sequential picture of change over a period of time has to a large extent precluded conceptual digressions on more general points at issue.

Thus, despite the obvious implications of this study for such general areas of sociological inquiry as the social psychology of health and illness, the complementarities and strains in family-hospital relations, the nature of identity change in the family, and the social genesis of deviance, it has not been expedient to develop these implications in their own right. Although allusion is made to them here and there, full discussion has had to be set aside in deference to narrational continuity. In the remaining pages, I should like to consider several of these implications for whatever light they may cast on continuing and emerging issues in current sociology.

THE SOCIAL PSYCHOLOGY OF HEALTH AND ILLNESS

At several places in this book, we have pointed out the influence of popular, commonsensical beliefs concerning health and illness on the family's reaction to the onset of the child's illness, on their attitudes toward his treatment and hospitalization, and on what they did and failed to do by way of implementing the rehabilitation prescriptions of the hospital. Thus, at the onset stage, for example, we saw how, for both good and bad, practical and injudicious reasons, the families tended to act as their own diagnosticians and therapists—that is, until such time as the child's condition could no longer be rationalized in terms of the lay diagnoses they had made. Later, during the long period of hospitalization, we traced the halting and circuitous process by which they came to adjust their layman's conceptions of time and progress in recovery so that it more nearly, although never wholly, accorded with those of the hospital. Still later, when the handicapped child returned home, we saw how difficult and frustrating it was for the family to accept and act upon the necessarily modest rehabilitational goals held out by medical authorities, and how for the most part they could conceive only of a "cure" or its absence.

These findings, along with strikingly similar ones from a variety of recent studies,[1] have important implications for both conceptual focus and strategy of research in the field of medical sociology. First, and most obviously, they point to the need for viewing health behavior in a social context much broader than that circumscribed by the consulting room, the clinic, and the hospital. The fact is that a considerable portion of the individual's health and illness experience takes place in locales and with persons far removed from the guidance and control of institutionalized medical authority—in the home, at work, with kin, friends, neighbors, and others in the person's routine orbit of

[1] E.g., Earl L. Koos, *The Health of Regionville,* New York: Columbia University Press, 1954; Eliot Freidson, *Patients' Views of Medical Practice,* New York: Russell Sage Foundation, 1961; Elaine Cumming and John Cumming, *Closed Ranks,* Cambridge: Harvard University Press, 1957.

existence. This is not to deny the strategic role of medical authority in many, though far from all, instances of illness. As we have seen, however, many other influences not only have an important bearing on when and how medical care is sought, but also support, negate, or otherwise modify the prescriptions and regimens dispensed by those officially charged with the patient's treatment and care.[2]

In addition to furthering a more realistic appreciation of the patient's situation, broadening the nexus of inquiry would also have significant bearing on the formulation of the medical sociologist's research problems. This stems from the circumstance that when the social researcher is presented with a problem in health behavior by the doctor, the nurse, the hospital administrator, or others strategically located in the official treatment system, he is likely to be offered what is, perhaps necessarily, a partial and value-weighted definition of the problem. What is it about the personality or social background of certain patients that makes them uncooperative? How can patients be persuaded to pay their bills on time, with less protest and sense of financial injury? Why don't more families follow through on recommended treatment for their children when it is obviously in their best interests to do so?

Given this kind of statement of the problem, the investigator runs the risk of structuring his inquiry so that it uncritically or unwittingly accords with the institutionally biased values and perspectives implicit in the very terms of the statement. He then seeks the cause of the problem in the patient or his family, neglecting the possibility that it may reside equally, or even primarily, in the socially patterned divergence of interests and outlooks in the patient-practitioner interaction.[3] Put more concretely, what is defined as problematic behavior by the doctor, for example, may from the patient's standpoint represent a rational and meaningful response to the expectations and sentiments of various significant persons in his environment. The reverse may be equally true; but, since it is unlikely that the medical sociologist will be consulted by patients for help in their problems with "unco-

[2] This and related points are extensively developed by Freidson, *op. cit.*

[3] The most definitive statement of this issue is by Julius Roth, "The Social Science Study of Medical Treatment," paper read at the Fifty-second Annual Meeting of the American Sociological Association, 1957.

operative" or "difficult" doctors, this side of the coin seldom receives attention.

Underlying these points is the more fundamental issue of the scope and guardianship of health values in our society. Few would question the pre-eminence accorded these values in contemporary America; their importance perhaps rivals attachment to material success and achievement. Indeed, the extraordinarily high repute and influence of the medical profession and its allied institutions derive in considerable measure from their safeguarding of values that nearly all classes of men invest with great significance. A common error, however, particularly on the part of those specialist groups charged with the guardianship and furtherance of these values, is to underestimate the concurrent attractiveness of other social values in the lives of men: e.g., wealth, power, love, prestige, knowledge, beauty, security, acceptance. As men attempt to realize simultaneously a plurality of values, innumerable occasions are bound to arise when the value of health, as it is represented by medical science, comes in conflict with, or fails to accommodate conveniently, the pursuit of one or more other values. And it is by no means obvious, necessary, or advisable that men will invariably resolve such conflicts wholly, or even partially, in favor of the health value. Here, as in many other areas of life, compromises and an ambivalent balancing-off of interests will usually be struck.

Ultimately, it is from this vantage point that much of what are viewed, often condescendingly, as popular, lay, or folk health practices are to be understood. Their existence signifies more than a vestigial, largely maladaptive cultural survival from an earlier, benighted social era; more than that which can easily be dismissed as "mere ignorance" or patronizingly explained away as the "exotic beliefs" of incompletely assimilated ethnic and class subcultures in our society. Taken in large, these are the patterned social responses of laymen to the many problematic issues that confront them as they try to calculate the advantages, costs, inconveniences, and benefits that may (or may not) accrue from consulting and heeding medical authority.

In weighing, therefore, the manner and frequency with which these "folk" beliefs, attitudes, and practices depart from and vitiate the diagnoses and prescriptions of medical authority, we would do well to consider the relevance of such departures for the more inclusive schemes of aspirations, expectations, and constraints by which men live. If this were done, we would find, I suspect, that what for the practitioner signifies an ignorant or anachronistic departure from approved health practice often represents for the layman a pragmatic and far from unreasonable compromise among his many, frequently conflicting, interests, engagements, and responsibilities. In short, it is not that laymen are necessarily unaware of, indifferent to, or hostile to the prescriptions of medical authority but, rather, that these cannot always be integrated economically with all else that engages them.

Certainly there will be occasions, usually of an extreme kind, when official health directives will be given absolute precedence over all else that concerns the layman. But, from his viewpoint, such directives are seldom so frequent, exigent, or unambiguous as the practitioner is wont to make them. It is because this difference of perspective exists that what are called lay conceptions of health also exist.

HOME AND HOSPITAL

The foregoing remarks touch closely on another issue that has concerned us in this book—the relationship of home and hospital. On the one side, we have seen how successful the hospital was in the important work of motivating the paralyzed child to ambulate again; how, within a relatively short time, it changed him from an acutely homesick child to someone who could tolerate, and even enjoy, the new and unfamiliar round of life that his treatment and long confinement entailed; how it provided him with a society of peers whose special standards and outlooks he learned to share so that he could then meaningfully relate his abnormal life situation to the particularistic aims of the therapeutic regime. On the other side, we have also seen how the hospital loosened the child's affective ties with home; how it induced behavioral changes in him that subsequently made his reincorporation into the home difficult and stressful for the family; how, most of all, it reacted with insensitivity and indifference to the parents' search for information, failing to give them an adequate understanding of the disease and its implications for the child's recovery and rehabilitation.

Could the first set of consequences have resulted without the second? Could the hospital and home have accommodated each other so fully that no untoward consequences, other than those wrought by the illness itself, would have ensued for either?

It would be rash to attempt a categorical answer to this question, if only because, as in all social relations, the degrees of freedom available to the respective parties vary so greatly from issue to issue. Thus, as regards the loosening of the child's affective ties with home, it would seem that the intense motivational demands made on the child by the physiotherapeutic regime could only be sustained in a specialized, non-homelike milieu, such as the hospital. (This supposition is partially borne out by the failure of many families to provide an adequate program of physiotherapy for the child once he returned home.) Because the success of this regime is based on more than mere rote application—rather, on a close identification of child with physiotherapist and on the moral support of other handicapped children similarly situated—it is probably unavoidable that the child will, temporarily at least, transfer certain of his attachments and loyalties from family to hospital.

Another largely unavoidable dilemma underlies those hospital-induced changes in the behavior of the child (greater demandingness, possessiveness, egocentrism) that later proved such a source of discord in the family. Even assuming, for the sake of argument, that the hospital were able to command much greater resources in time, personnel, and equipment than it currently can—and, further, that its patient-care policies were unusually liberal and psychologically supportive in their design and implementation—there would still remain, for example, a marked qualitative difference in what a nurse must do to manage a large group of children on a ward compared with what a mother can do with her own child in her own home. The reasons for this are too numerous and obvious to list here. Suffice it to say that, because of certain irreducible dissimilarities in the two situations, the child on the ward will of necessity learn to attend to normative rules and expectations different from those applying at home. When he returns to the family, it will not be easy for him immediately to discard the crude equalitarian norms that for the most part governed his relationships in the hospital in favor of the more flexible and diffuse norms of family living.

Here again, what is functional for the hospital treatment system leads to certain dysfunctional consequences for the family interactional system. But, given the distinctive goals, resource requirements, and organizational features of the two systems, it is doubtful that much can be done to resolve this dilemma.

Fortunately, not all issues that arise between family and hospital are subject to so little freedom of choice and resolution. We have indicated that the hospital might have done much more than it actually did in communicating information to the family about the disease and the child's prospects for recovery; in motivating the parents to implement in the home the rehabilitational program prescribed for the child; and, last though far from least, in preparing them psychologically for the many emotional and social problems they were bound to encounter as a result of existing prejudices toward the visibly handicapped. Although one can trace the institutional and psychological sources of resistance, on the part of both family and hospital, to attempts to communicate fully and frankly, it should be recognized that there is nothing intrinsic in the family-hospital relationship that absolutely precludes such attempts. On the contrary, it can be argued that providing systematically for them would represent a significant step toward realizing the basic ideals and practical ends of medical intervention.

How, then, can the hospital undertake these tasks more effectively? Without going into highly specific policy and organizational issues, there certainly seems a need for a broader definition of therapeutic activity by treatment personnel. Such a definition would not be confined to the routine, neatly bounded tasks of diagnosis, prescription, and physical treatment but would seek to embrace in addition the many problematic issues of communication, motivation, and social circumstance that also play a part in the state of the patient's health and in the meaning his illness has for him and his family. Although explicit modifications in the treatment policies and therapeutic philosophy of a hospital can in themselves do much toward making such a definition operative, its practical realization ultimately depends more on the values, understandings, and skills acquired by treatment staff members (doctors, nurses, physiotherapists, occupational therapists) during the course of their professional training. It is reassuring that educators in the health professions are coming more and more to appreciate the social and psychological dimensions of treatment, care, and rehabilitation. Although this appreciation was not yet evidenced in the treatment and care dispensed to the children and families in this study, it augurs well for the humane quality of hospital practice in the future.

Beyond this, to the degree that present-day treatment staff is unable, by reason of earlier training, occupational temperament, or work load, to attend to the many contextual issues of a socio-emotional kind that impinge on the patient, it is incumbent on hospital authorities to utilize as fully and imaginatively as possible the services of other professional workers whose training, we can assume, more nearly fits them for this task: e.g., the medical and psychiatric social worker, the family counselor, the parent group worker.[4] The proper integration of these specialists into the hospital structure would not only make for a broadened, more humane definition of the therapeutic task but would also help to ameliorate at least some of the secondary social stresses and disruptions now occasioned by serious illness and hospitalization. That many otherwise modern and well-run hospitals have failed to provide for these services testifies less, in this writer's opinion, to the existence of inherent or insuperable obstacles than it does to short-sightedness in their underlying conception of the patient and his problems.

To bring together the strands of this discussion, we would hold that some of the stresses and disturbances in family life occasioned by prolonged treatment and hospitalization can be avoided, but that others probably cannot. The avoidable ones are those which, in the main, derive from various of the hospital's institutionalized, though often unintended, evasions of the basic, historically sanctioned terms of the therapist-patient relationship—such evasions as the failure to

[4] Neither of the two convalescent hospitals dealt with in this study employed a single full-time social worker. At one there was a less-than-half-time worker; at the other a worker was called in only "when needed," on the average of one afternoon a month. Despite their problems in obtaining information from the doctor and in disciplining the handicapped child, it was never arranged for any of the parents in this study to consult a social worker or other kind of family counselor. In walking through the plant of these same hospitals, however, one sees vast amounts of little-used and obsolete orthopedic and physiotherapeutic equipment that must represent a sizable capital investment.

communicate relevant information about the patient's condition to him and his family, the failure to provide for adequate continuity of treatment, and the failure to be receptive to the socio-emotional meanings of illness—in sum, the oft-noted failure to approach the patient as person, not solely as diseased object.

The unavoidable stresses are those which, on the whole, are more closely linked to such relatively unalterable circumstances as the fact of illness itself, the temporary or long-term dismemberment of the family unit, the restrictions and special social demands placed on the patient for the purpose of helping him to get well, and, in the last analysis, the impossibility that any hospital setting can duplicate for the patient, or even crudely approximate, his life situation at home. Whether this or that aspect of treatment or hospitalization "is really necessary" can, of course, always be argued; but, regardless of the generosity or severity of policy with respect to such matters, enough adheres to the bald circumstances of illness and hospitalization to make for anguish and disruption in the family.

These remarks comprise a more detailed statement of the theme enunciated in the introduction to this book; namely, that hospital and family are, and must of necessity remain, distinct types of organization, each with its own purposes, procedures, and requirements. Although each is capable of sufficient flexibility to successfully accommodate the other in some areas, in other areas their needs and interests diverge so sharply as to produce strain.

CHANGE AND CONTINUITY OF IDENTITY IN THE FAMILY

Throughout this work we have been concerned with the way in which the child and his family came to conceive of themselves as a result of the child's illness, his separation from the home, and his reincorporation into it as a handicapped person. The data appear to suggest a striking anomaly: although it is clear that much was changed in the family, both objectively and subjectively, by these experiences, it is equally clear that the appreciation by family members of what had transpired in no way matched the magnitude of the changes themselves. Regardless of whether, for example, the families normalized or disassociated the social meaning of the child's handicap, the ebb and flow of daily life appeared to remain sufficiently static to leave them with the conviction that nothing had changed, that the child was essentially the same person he had been prior to his illness, and that everyone in the family felt and acted toward the others as he always had.

It is less important to question the accuracy of such perceptions—that they contradicted certain of the existential realities has been amply documented—than it is to weigh their significance for the organizational stability and psychological continuity of family life. For, as was suggested in Chapter 6, the disparity between the changes actually wrought and their reflexive effects on family identity is at the very heart of the question of how a corporate entity such as the family can, in the face of the unexpected, the disruptive, and the transforming, continue to function without breaking drastically from its particular historic identity. Many factors contributed to this accomplishment; two of them we shall review here for whatever they may suggest about the general requirements for stable functioning and continuity of identity in the contemporary family.

Certainly, one of the more obvious factors has to do with the sheer structural dynamics of the crisis itself. By this I mean that, had it been a parent rather than a child who was stricken, it is much less likely that the families could have entertained the conviction that "nothing had really changed." Many of the more central functions of family life—breadwinning, child care, housekeeping, sex, recreation—would have been so vitally disrupted as to make it exceedingly difficult for the family subsequently to reconstruct the experience so that it "fit in," psychologically speaking, with a known past and an imagined future. But because the stricken member was a child and not a parent, these vital functions, while by no means unaffected, retained sufficient integrity to permit the family to assimilate the experience into the familiar modalities of their existence. Moreover, because it was a child, and because childhood is so distinctively vested with an aura of futurity, it was possible both theoretically and actually for the families to suspend judgment, as it were, on the question of the long-term significance of his handicap. This afforded ample time and good reason to experiment *in vivo* with the favored proposition that, despite important alterations in their own lives and in the child's chances for realizing the fully "normal" life they prized for him, nothing had "really" changed. Hence the future, it was thought, could unfold in the salutary way in which they had always imagined it would.

To say that these primary functions remained largely intact is also to imply that the daily round of life of the family retained much of its pre-crisis focus, rhythm, and ambience. This too, made for continuity of identity and, hence, for the maintenance of those core understandings, sentiments, and practices by which the family customarily regulated its group life. One has only to consider the many props and pursuits of daily existence that retained their familiar qualities to appreciate how unlikely it would have been for these families to be engulfed by anomie or some other disorganized state. Thus, for example, the husband went to work much as he always had; the wife typically had other children to look after and the usual household chores to do; the children went to school, played, and fought in their familiar way; furniture, house, and neighborhood retained their recognizable properties, as did friends, relatives, and neighbors; the family standard of living was not altered significantly, for better or worse.

This is not to say that these aspects of daily life remained untouched by the polio child's illness, separation from home, and physical disability; indeed, much of this book has been devoted to showing how they were affected by what happened. But demonstrating that they were affected, even significantly so, is completely different from claiming that there also resulted a sudden or considered alteration in the family's fundamental sense of who and what they were and what their collective life meant to them—that is, a discontinuity of identity. It is precisely the failure of the latter to follow from the former that is so intriguing and noteworthy about these families, particularly those in which the child sustained a more than minor handicap.

Metaphorically, this phenomenon may be likened to a fleetingly glimpsed, occasionally distracting repair in an elaborate tapestry— enough of the fabric of family life remained intact to make what was new and different in the weave blend in (albeit incongruously, from certain angles and in certain lights) with the familiar design of the whole. Or, as in the figure-ground problem in Gestalt psychology, the ground—here, the existential aggregate of family pursuits, interests, and relations—retained enough of its contour and detail so that the alteration in the figure—i.e., the new situation brought into being by the child's handicap—failed to induce a perceptual reorganization of the total field.

THE STUDY OF DEVIANCE

In recent years a more sophisticated approach to the study of deviance has become evident in social science. The works of Lemert, Becker, Cohen, Cloward, and Goffman[5] have been in the forefront of a growing number of attempts to view this phenomenon from a broader, less parochial perspective, one in which deviance and deviant processes are treated as integral parts of the functioning of institutions and social structures. Prior to this, and even today, the predominant orientation in American social science has been to regard deviance almost exclusively in terms of the pathological, the abnormal, the psychologically unstable—at best, as an unwholesome, though perhaps unwilling, departure from social norms. In line with this conception, the tendency of countless researches in this field, on subjects ranging from breakfast-food choices to bureaucratic decision-making, has been to search for the roots of deviance in such entities as basic personality, childhood experience, and unconscious motivation.

Irrespective of the possible relevance of such entities to the genesis of deviance, it is to the credit of the writers mentioned above that they have shifted the topic away from a predominantly pathological locus to a level at which it is conceived as a constituent element in social process—a ubiquitous, and perhaps necessary, accompaniment to group life.[6] Hence, it becomes possible to see deviant processes where previously one saw only the "deviant," to conceive of deviant phases, contingencies, and episodes in the lives and careers of even the

[5] Edwin M. Lemert, *Social Pathology,* New York: McGraw-Hill, 1951; Howard S. Becker, *Outsiders,* Glencoe, Ill.: Free Press, in press; Albert K. Cohen, *Delinquent Boys,* Glencoe, Ill.: Free Press, 1955; Richard A. Cloward and Lloyd E. Ohlin, *Delinquency and Opportunity,* Glencoe, Ill.: Free Press, 1960; Erving Goffman, *Asylums,* New York: Doubleday Anchor, 1961.

[6] Cf. Robert A. Dentler and Kai T. Erikson, "The Functions of Deviance in Groups," *Social Problems,* VII, 2 (Fall, 1959), 98-107.

most conforming of "normals." This widening of intellectual horizons on so important an issue can do much to redress the scarcely hidden bias implicit in so much previous work and thought in the field; it may even result in transferring some of the onus for the individual's deviance away from the encapsulated psyche of the psychiatric case history and personality profile of the projective test report.

Although the present study does not deal primarily with problems commonly thought of as falling in this area, it may throw some light on the question of how one set of persons, with no prior history of deviance, came to be viewed, and to view themselves, as deviant, as a result of an accident of physiology and the social reactions elicited by its effects on the body. At least as far as the nine handicapped children in this group were concerned, "deviance" from "normality" had in the beginning markedly less to do with their own wishes, attitudes, and fears than it did with the persons and social arrangements they confronted daily. It was mainly through this disjunction in their own and others' perceptions of them that they were being exposed to certain differential experiences and associations that, it can be assumed, would in time result in their acquiring identities distinctly different from those possessed by their "normal" peers. The resultant "deviance" that later in their lives might be interpreted in terms of some personality trait or aberration of childhood upbringing could, it would seem, be more accurately accounted for by those very processes in which the handicapped child comes to be socially categorized as "different."

While it would be dogmatic to maintain that all deviance is of this order, it may not be amiss to note that it takes at least two to make a "deviant"—the actor and the beholder. To grant this little is to grant the presence of a significant societal component in all that is labeled deviance, from the most bizarre to the most institutionalized. The task of sociology, therefore, is to assess constantly and tenaciously the scope and *raison d'être* of this component and to determine how much it, by itself, fashions the "deviance" seen in the individual. If nothing else, the study of deviance from this perspective can tell us as much about the society that so categorizes certain acts as it can about the individuals who perform them.

APPENDIX A

Study Background, Population, and Methods

The data for this study derive from a much more extensive inter-disciplinary project begun in 1953 at the Psychiatric Institute of the University of Maryland Medical School. The staff of that project, on which I served in the capacity of sociologist, included, in addition, two psychologists, a child psychiatrist, a psychiatric social worker, and a pediatrician. The project had as its general aim the comprehensive investigation of all the factors—psychological, social, and physiolog-ical—involved in the perception of and adjustment to the experience of paralytic polio by a selected group of children and their families. Toward this end, a voluminous body of interview, observational, test, and medical data was collected from them over a three-year period. It is estimated, for example, that an average of fifty hours of interview-ing time alone was spent with each family. Ten of the families were first seen by the project staff during the late summer and fall of 1954, and the remaining four were brought into the research approximately a year later. Of these 14, only one family, the Stewarts, withdrew from the study prior to its scheduled termination date.[1]

[1] This occurred approximately a year after the family came into the study. Mrs. Stewart gave as her reason for withdrawing that she, her husband, and daughter found the interviews with the project staff upsetting; that the questions asked reminded them of events and thoughts of which they would rather not be reminded.

THE FAMILIES

The inclusion of a family in the larger study first depended, of course, on a child from that family's contracting the paralytic variety of poliomyelitis. The other criteria of selection used were, in general, designed to ensure a certain degree of homogeneity among cases and representativeness with respect to the major pathological and epidemiological characteristics of the disease. These criteria were as follows:

1. That the stricken child be between four and twelve years of age. (This group accounted for roughly 65 per cent of paralytic-polio incidence in the metropolitan area of Baltimore.)

2. That he have spinal paralytic poliomyelitis and not the more uncommon bulbar or encephalitic forms. (Spinal poliomyelitis accounted for roughly 70 per cent of paralytic-polio incidence.)

3. That the major site of paralysis be the lower extremities. (Primary lower-extremity involvement accounted for more than 50 per cent of children left paralyzed by polio.)

4. That the child be white. (Comprising roughly 27 per cent of the population of the Baltimore area, Negroes accounted for only 15 per cent of its polio incidence.)

5. That he come from a "clinically normal" home—i.e., that he not be a foster child or resident in some institution and that at least the mother be living.

Although it might have been desirable to include in the research design such additional criteria of selection as severity of disease involvement, socioeconomic status, and ethnic origin, any attempt to do so would have reduced the already small number of cases to a mere handful. As finally constituted, the study population of 14 consisted of ten working-class and four lower-middle-class families. The group included eight Protestant Anglo-Saxons, two second-generation Jewish families, two Catholic families, and two families of mixed Catholic-Protestant affiliation.[2]

[2] See Appendix B for a more detailed inventory of the social characteristics of the 14 families.

THE RESEARCH METHODS

A wide variety of research instruments and approaches was used in studying the children and their families.

Interviews with Parents

Periodic open-ended interviews were held with the mother of each child, including one very lengthy interview devoted to gathering a social history of the family. These interviews averaged an hour in length. Typically, fourteen such contacts were made during the eighteen- to twenty-four-month period in which the families were seen. The interviews were scheduled so as to correspond as much as possible with the natural course of the disease and its treatment. That is, the first interview was conducted within a week of the child's admission to the pediatrics ward of the receiving hospital; at least three interviews, but usually four or five, were conducted during the child's two- to seven-month stay in the convalescent hospital; on the average, ten contacts were made, at increasing time intervals, during the year or so following the child's discharge from the convalescent hospital.

At least two open-ended interviews were conducted with the father of each child, the first within a week of the child's admission to the acute polio ward and the second when the family was last seen. In about half the families, circumstances permitted more frequent interviews with the father.

With a few exceptions, all interviews with parents were tape-recorded and later transcribed in full. Except for some four or five interviews with one family, all the parent interviews were conducted by the psychiatric social worker or the sociologist, each assuming continuing responsibility for seven of the sets of parents.

Interviews with and Tests of the Children

The project's child psychiatrist conducted an average of fifteen free, unstructured interviews, each approximately half an hour long, with each child. Where appropriate, such approaches as doll play, game play, drawing, and finger painting were utilized. Although these interviews with the children were visual in content to a large extent, the verbal portions were recorded and later transcribed.

Three to five sessions, each of roughly forty-five minutes' duration, were devoted to a psychological examination of each child. Such projective techniques as the Children's Apperception Test, the Rorschach, and human figure drawings were used. These instruments were administered by one of the project's psychologists.

A periodic physical examination of each child, usually of half an hour's duration, was conducted by the project's pediatrician. On the average, eight to ten such examinations were made during the eighteen- to twenty-four-month period. Their purpose was primarily to determine the amount and type of polio-caused muscle damage sustained by each child and to estimate, in this connection, his functional capacities.

Like the parent interviews, the contacts with the children were phased so as to correspond as closely as possible with the course of the disease and its treatment.

Other Data Sources

A series of partially open-ended but mainly schedule-type interviews was held with hospital personnel (doctors, nurses, physiotherapists, occupational therapists, hospital schoolteachers) charged with the treatment and care of each child during his confinement in the admission and convalescent hospitals. These interviews were intended to elicit information concerning the child's physical state, psychological condition, and behavior in the wards. They were conducted by the child psychiatrist, psychiatric social worker, and sociologist. Apart from the specific information that they furnished on each child, these interviews were a highly valuable source of data on the role behavior and professional attitudes of the various classes of treatment personnel.

At various times, in various connections, observations were made and noted by all the project workers of the children on the ward as they underwent examination and participated in physiotherapy sessions and other activities around the hospital. These provided an over-all view of hospital routine and practices in the management of acute and convalescent polio cases.

A comprehensive series of interviews was held with persons trained and experienced in one or more phases of the diagnosis, treatment, care, and rehabilitation of polio patients. Included in this group were orthopedic surgeons, physical-medicine specialists, physiotherapists, pediatricians, and a wide cross-section of welfare workers concerned in one way or another with polio patients and their families—e.g., vocational rehabilitation officers, National Foundation personnel, counselors and directors of camps for the handicapped, and school officials in charge of specialized programs for handicapped children.

Use of Data

From this vast and, frankly, somewhat unassimilable collection of data, by far the major sources utilized throughout this book were the interviews with the parents. In the sections dealing with the recovery perspectives of the families (Chapters 3 and 4), considerable use was also made of the interviews with treatment personnel and of the observational notes on hospital routines and practices. Only very minor and incidental use was made of the sizable body of unstructured psychiatric-type interviews with the children and of their responses on the many psychological projective tests administered to them. The decision to utilize these materials only incidentally was based on several considerations: First, these data are extremely diffuse and, in their manifest content, at least, rarely addressed to the central questions of this study. Secondly, as a sociologist, I was not equipped to analyze them in accordance with the purposes for which they had been collected—i.e., depth psychological interpretations of the child's personality and current psychic state. Thirdly, the inevitable limitations of time and energy in the face of the project's vast accumulation of all varieties of data necessitated certain arbitrary decisions concerning which data to include.

Although a very large portion of the available data was excluded, it would be false to claim that anything approximating a formal, exhaustive content analysis was attempted with the extensive body of data I did use. (The parent interviews alone add up to some five thousand pages of typescript.) This analysis could better be described as the final product of a long process of rumination that bridged several years of active participation in the formulation of the project's research design and objectives, in the collection of data, and in the preliminary evaluation of themes and trends contained therein. Throughout this period I formulated and reformulated, untold times, the basic questions to which I eventually applied the data. Only when these questions had crystallized sufficiently in my mind did I systematically go through the whole accumulation of project data, choosing and discarding, excerpting, abstracting, and comparing them for what light they would throw on the problems I had marked off for study.

APPENDIX B

Social Characteristics of the 14 Families

Name	Age[1]	Yrs. of School Completed by Parents[1]	Religion	Occupation of Parent (s)	Socio-economic level of Family[2]
Mr. Baker	30	14	Baptist	Junior engineer for large firm	Middle class
Mrs. Baker	28	13	Baptist		
*Gerald	6				
Jim	3				
Mr. Eaton	33	11	Baptist	Carpenter	Working class
Mrs. Eaton	30	9	Baptist		
*Geraldine	11				
Henry	7				
Tom	2				
Alice Sue	1 mo.				
Mr. Ellsworth	28	14	Baptist	Traffic manager, studying to become teacher	Middle class
Mrs. Ellsworth	30	16	Episcopalian	Librarian	
*Sarah	5½				
Mr. Harris	34	10	Jewish	Loan-company collector	Lower middle class
Mrs. Harris	32	10	Jewish		
*Marvin	11				
Keith	4½				

[1] Ages of family members are those at time of child's admission to hospital.
[2] Classification is based on Hollingshead's *Index of Social Position Score*. Families designated as working class are the equivalent of his Classes IV and V; those designated as lower-middle and middle, the equivalent of his Classes III and II, respectively. See A. B. Hollingshead and F. C. Redlich, *Social Class and Mental Illness*, New York: Wiley, 1958, pp. 387-97.

* Denotes child with poliomyelitis.

Name	Age		Religion	Occupation	Class
Mr. Johnson	28	9	Baptist	Assembly-line worker in aircraft plant	Working class
Mrs. Johnson	26	11	Baptist	Part-time sales clerk	
*Richard	7				
Kenneth	5				
Raymond	3				
Barbara	6 mo.				
Mr. Lawson	29	11	Catholic	Manager of small hardware store	Working class
Mrs. Lawson	28	9	Catholic		
*John	8				
Marie	7				
Henry	5				
Francis	3				
Thomas	6 mo.				
Mr. Lee	32	7	Baptist	Unemployed welder, longshoreman	Working class
Mrs. Lee	27	8	Baptist		
Paul	9				
*Frank	4½				
Mr. Manning	32	12	Methodist	Steel-mill machinist	Working class
Mrs. Manning	30	8	Catholic	Part-time supermarket cashier	
*Polly	6½				
Eunice	3				
Mr. Mason	45	7	Baptist	Lumber-mill foreman	Working class
Mrs. Mason	41	8	Lutheran		
Roger	23				
Neil	18				
*Norma Jean	9				

* Denotes child with poliomyelitis.

continued on page 190

APPENDIX B (cont.)

Social Characteristics of the 14 Families

Name	Age[1]	Yrs. of School Completed by Parents	Religion	Occupation of Parent (s)	Socio-economic level of Family[2]
Mr. Paulus	28	10	Catholic	Lathe operator	Working class
Mrs. Paulus	30	12	Presbyterian	Part-time department-store sales clerk	
*Laura	6				
Joseph	2				
Mr. Prince	32	11	Jewish	Bakery-truck driver	Working class
Mrs. Prince	29	12	Jewish	Part-time beautician's helper	
Harold	9½				
*David	5				
Mr. Richards	28	12	Baptist	Furniture-warehouse dispatcher	Working class
Mrs. Richards	25	12	Baptist		
*Neil	6				
Donald	5				
Mr. Short	31	14	Methodist	Bank teller	Lower middle class
Mrs. Short	26	10	Methodist		
*Edward	7				
Connie	2				
Mr. Stewart	36	8	Catholic	Plant guard	Working class
Mrs. Stewart	31	8	Catholic		
*Theresa	12				

[1] Ages of family members are those at time of child's admission to hospital.

[2] Classification is based on Hollingshead's *Index of Social Position Score*. Families designated as working class are the equivalent of his Classes IV and V; those designated as lower-middle and middle, the equivalent of his Classes III and II, respectively. See A. B. Hollingshead and F. C. Redlich, *Social Class and Mental Illness*, New York: Wiley, 1958, pp. 387-97.

* Denotes child with poliomyelitis.

INDEX

191